the
real
food
diet
COOKBOOK

Copyright © 2011 by Exodus Health Center LLC
The Library of Congress cataloging-in-publication data
Axe, Josh
The Real Food Diet Cookbook: Delicious Real Recipes
for Losing Weight, Feeling Great, and Transforming
your Health / Dr. Josh Axe
ISBN 978-0-615-38666-9 (hardcover)
1. Health 2. Nutrition 3. Cooking

Printed in USA.

This book may be purchased for business, educational, or sales promotional use. For information or to order, please contact:

Exodus Health Center
15123 Old Hickory Blvd
Nashville, TN 37211
615-445-7701
615-445-7771 (fax)
www.draxe.com

ISBN-13:   978-0-615-38666-9
ISBN-10:   0-615-38666-0

Editor-in-Chief: Jennifer Lill
Project Manager: Lori Winter
Contributing Editor: Leslie Parker
Cover Design: Drew Winter
Interior Design: Mary Hooper/Milkglass Creative
Photographers: Allison Hendrickson and Don Wright

the
real
food
diet
COOKBOOK

Dr. Josh Axe

the real food diet cookbook

"The health status of America today is very bleak. With more than two-thirds of adults now overweight or obese, nearly half of the population at risk of heart disease, and more than one in three people diagnosed with cancer in their lifetimes, people are desperate for a new hope. With multiplied millions suffering from diabetes, autism, Alzheimer's, Parkinson's disease, and the explosion of immune, digestive and inflammatory disorders, it's clear we need a nationwide health transformation. Combining ancient wisdom with modern science, Dr. Josh Axe and his *Real Food Diet Cookbook* can provide a roadmap to take your health to the next level. With delicious and simple recipes containing many of your favorite ingredients, *The Real Food Diet Cookbook* can provide optimal nutrition for the entire family. If you want to reduce allergies, boost your energy, improve your mood, shrink your waistline, and supercharge your immune system, then it's time you began the Real Food Diet!"

JORDAN RUBIN, NMD, PHD
Founder of Garden of Life, New York Times Bestselling Author of *The Maker's Diet*

"When it comes to changing our lifestyle, we need a "how-to" book, and *The Real Food Diet Cookbook* is the one to keep close by to guide us everyday. We live in a toxic world, and Dr. Axe teaches us how to fix it from the inside out, starting with what we put in our bodies! We need to know what foods are inflammatory, what foods are healing, and what foods prevent disease. Dr. Josh Axe not only guides us through the ingredients, but he has delicious, practical recipes and menus to guide us to better care for ourselves and our families."

DANIEL B. KALB, MD, MPH, FAAFP
Cool Springs Family Medicine

"Message received! Dr. Axe's cookbook drives home the fact that you CAN have it all. In a time when many people think eating right is synonymous with eating food with no flavor, Dr. Axe brings us what we thought was a food paradox: savory, beautiful, and... HEALTHY! Simple selections to prepare, yet difficult tastes to beat, these meals can help you lower inflammation, boost immune function, and optimize metabolism. It's all in this book. Well done!"

MICHAEL R. BERNUI, D.O., FAAFP
Founder and Medical Director of the Center for Restorative Medicine

acknowledgements

I wish to thank all the people who have inspired me through the task of writing this book:

To my parents, Gary and Winona, whose love for me taught me to love other people well.

I would also like to recognize my brother Jordan and give a special thanks to my sister Rachel who has been with me from the beginning.

Thanks to Jennifer Lill, my brilliant partner in writing this book. You are a visionary, helped me laugh, and made the process fun.

Thanks to my personal assistant Lori Winter. Without you, my whole world would fall apart.

To Mary Hooper for your creative spirit and artistic ability.

To Drew Winter for your thoughts and work in design.

And thanks to Allison Hendrickson and Don Wright whose photos are works of art.

Thanks to my team at Exodus Health Center and my patients for having patience with me in getting this cookbook out!

A special thanks to Leslie Parker who helps run my world.

Thanks to many of the physicians who have inspired me to save lives.

A special thanks to my closest friend, Dr. Peter Camiolo. As they say, iron sharpens iron.

And finally, thanks to God for His unconditional love. He gave me hands to write and a mouth to speak the truth of health and healing. To Him be all glory and honor.

table of contents

recipes

breakfast

beverages

salads

snacks

desserts

food math 101

Ever heard of food math? Don't worry. Neither has anyone else. Why? It doesn't exist. But I'll use it here to illustrate a point:

$$\text{Atkins}^2 \div \text{Zone} \times {}^3/_8{}^\circ + (\sqrt{\text{Scarsdale}} \pm \pi)$$

$$\geq \quad \text{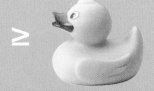} \quad \times \text{South Beach}^3$$

Confused? Well you should be...

With all the contradicting information out there, it seems impossible to find a food equation that is both simple and effective. What's healthy? What's not? All things in moderation? Some things in moderation? Carbs? Calories? Fat?

And we wonder why eating right seems so hard!

It may seem like rocket science, but it's not. Healthy cooking is not and never should be considered a fad—it's simply eating the way nature intended. By purchasing this cookbook, you have taken the first step in transforming your health, as well as your time in the kitchen.

This cookbook contains recipes with three things in mind:

You love food.　　　**You are busy.**　　　**You want to feel better and look better.**

My name is Dr. Josh Axe, and I love food, too. I used to be just like you. I thought eating healthy meant you had to eat sticks, grass, dried tuna, and Brussels sprouts. But I found that eating real, natural foods and using proper preparation can make food taste amazing.

And the added bonus, you are going to lose weight and feel great. I used to be the guy who ate nothing but chicken breast and dried out broccoli, and I thought that was eating right. I had a lot to learn. Eating the right foods doesn't have to be a chore. With the right recipes—like the ones in this book—you'll find out how delicious eating healthy can be.

This book is filled with short, easy recipes that taste amazing and will make you feel better. *What more could you ask for?* Remember, it's not rocket science.

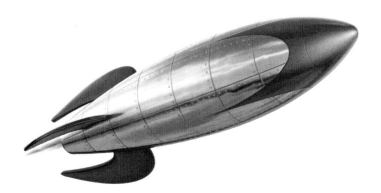

real food

vs.

fake food

Before we can learn how to transform our food, we have to learn the difference between the real stuff and the imposters.

imposters!

Real food is just what it sounds like: food in its most basic form taken directly from nature without additives, alterations, or fillers. So, what about fake food? When most people think of "fake food," they picture wax fruit sitting in a bowl. Unfortunately, fake food is actually food that we consume every day that's disguised as consumable food.

Don't blame the fake food. It started out with good intentions to nourish your body. So, where does fake food go wrong? And how does this happen? Here's an example:

Allow me to introduce the apple, which is perfect because it has almost everything your body needs. It's full of fiber, water, enzymes, vitamins, minerals, electrolytes, and antioxidants.

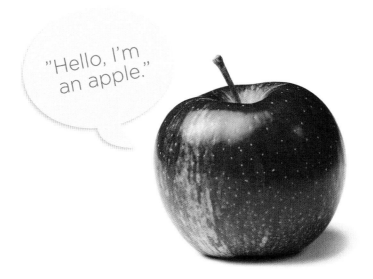

But that's when the process of turning a real food into a fake food begins.

We take this real food and remove its peel, which contains the majority of the antioxidants and fiber. Then we mash the poor, innocent fruit down and press it so that only the juice remains. We then take this juice and pasteurize it, which heats the juice at 150 degrees for 40 minutes, killing off all the nutrients. Next, we remove the water to make a concentrate. Then we decide to turn it back into juice again, and in pour the preservatives, tap water, coloring, and added sugar.

So, we started with a delicious and nutritious apple and ended up with glorified sugar water. This, my friends, is how a real food becomes a fake food.

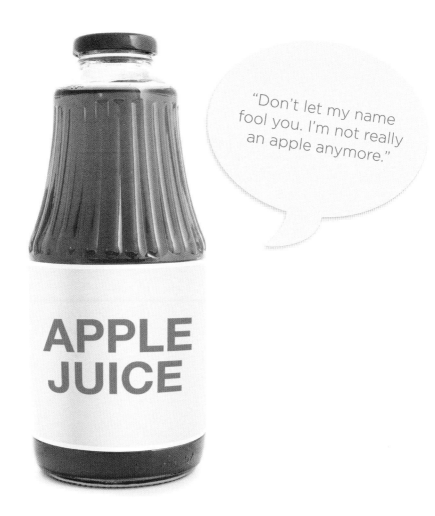

"Don't let my name fool you. I'm not really an apple anymore."

It's a little depressing when you look at the process on paper. Well, guess what? Our bodies think so, too. Our systems were made for real foods the way they are found in nature. Would you fuel your car with imitation gasoline? Well, if you wouldn't do that to your car, why would you do it to your body?

Apple - Fiber - Nutrients + Additives = FAKE FOOD

nutrient density

Now that we know how a real food becomes a fake food, let's discuss in a little more detail the "why" behind it all. It's a simple concept called Nutrient Density, and it's the reason why real food is ALWAYS better than fake food.

Nutrient Density (ND) is a way to classify the amount of nutrients in food, both real and fake. It's a scale that ranges from 0 to 1000, with 1000 being the most nutritious "super foods" (such as kale), and every other food falling somewhere in between.

What's surprising to many people is that the highest-ranking foods as far as nutrients are concerned are found not in whole grains, but in vegetables and fruits. For example, with a ND rating of 53 for oatmeal (a food traditionally considered "healthy") and a ND rating of 1000 for kale, it would literally require you to eat 20 bowls of oatmeal to match the nutrients found in 1 bowl of kale!

The Nutrient Density chart I have provided will show you where many of the most common foods fall in terms of nutrients. And it's obvious who wins in the battle between real and fake food. Real food is ALWAYS better because it's packed with vitamins, minerals, antioxidants, enzymes, and a host of other nutrients that are vital for a healthy body.

As the saying goes, Americans are overfed but undernourished. And let's face it. If your cells don't have nutrients, you are going to be sick. We obsess over counting calories, fats, and carbs, but we never count nutrients. It just doesn't make sense!

BOTTOM LINE:

Don't Count Calories, Count Nutrients!

top 30 nutrient dense foods

MY TOP 30 LIST OF NUTRITIOUS FOODS AND THEIR NUTRIENT SCORES

1.	COLLARD, MUSTARD, & TURNIP GREENS	11.	BEAN SPROUTS	21.	PLUM
	1,000		444		157
2.	KALE	12.	RED PEPPERS	22.	RASPBERRIES
	1,000		420		145
3.	WATERCRESS	13.	ROMAINE LETTUCE	23.	BLUEBERRIES
	1,000		389		130
4.	BOK CHOY	14.	BROCCOLI	24.	PAPAYA
	824		376		118
5.	SPINACH	15.	CARROT JUICE	25.	BRAZIL NUTS
	739		344		116
6.	BRUSSELS SPROUTS	16.	TOMATOES + TOMATO PROUCTS	26.	ORANGES
	672		90-300		109
7.	SWISS CHARD	17.	CAULIFLOWER	27.	APPLE
	670		295		72
8.	ARUGULA	18.	STRAWBERRIES	28.	BEANS, NOT CANNED (all varieties)
	559		212		55-70
9.	RADISH	19.	POMEGRANATE JUICE	29.	SEEDS: FLAXSEED, SUNFLOWER, SESAME
	554		193		45
10.	CABBAGE	20.	BLACKBERRIES	30.	WALNUTS
	481		178		29

* The Nutrient Density rating system was created by Dr. Joel Fuhrman to evaluate and compare the levels of vitamins, minerals, phytonutrients, and antioxidants found in our food.

the real food pyramid

If you've ever seen America's Standard Food Pyramid, you know that it recommends eating six to ten servings of grains and breads a day. Umm, okay. Have you ever actually eaten ten servings of bread a day and not woken up in a coma or ten pounds heavier??

Eating six to ten servings of grains is like eating 3 slices of pizza, 2 sandwiches, and a giant bowl of pasta in one day!

Does this really sound healthy to you? Anyone with common sense can understand that following the guidelines of the Standard Food Pyramid is going to make you sick.

That's why I've created the Real Food Pyramid. The Real Food Pyramid is focused on boosting your nutrient density and decreasing your blood glucose levels, which helps you lose weight and increase energy. And it works because it's based on getting more servings of the foods that have the most fiber, vitamins, minerals, antioxidants, protein, and healthy fats.

So, if you want to revolutionize your health, lose weight, reverse disease, and feel energy like you've never experienced...

DITCH THE

STANDARD FOOD PYRAMID

&

START FOLLOWING

THE REAL FOOD PYRAMID

THE REAL FOOD
PYRAMID

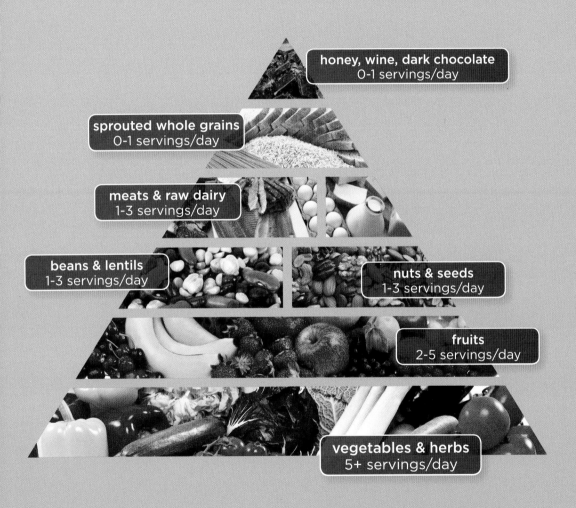

honey, wine, dark chocolate
0-1 servings/day

sprouted whole grains
0-1 servings/day

meats & raw dairy
1-3 servings/day

beans & lentils
1-3 servings/day

nuts & seeds
1-3 servings/day

fruits
2-5 servings/day

vegetables & herbs
5+ servings/day

check your baggage

Alright, we need to do a little mental housekeeping first. Get rid of all preconceptions about diet. Drown out the voices in your head chanting worn-out diet mantras and replace all that with one simple idea:

QUALITY OVER QUANTITY

Oh, you've heard that before? Of course you have! It's a cliché for a reason—because it's true. Perhaps with a few exceptions like money and hair, "quality over quantity" holds its weight, especially when it comes to food.

Stop counting calories.

Stop counting fat.

Stop counting carbs.

Stop measuring every last portion on your miniscale.

Start focusing on eating quality food.

Pretty soon, you will see that if you're eating the right stuff, counting calories and time consuming measuring will be a thing of the past.

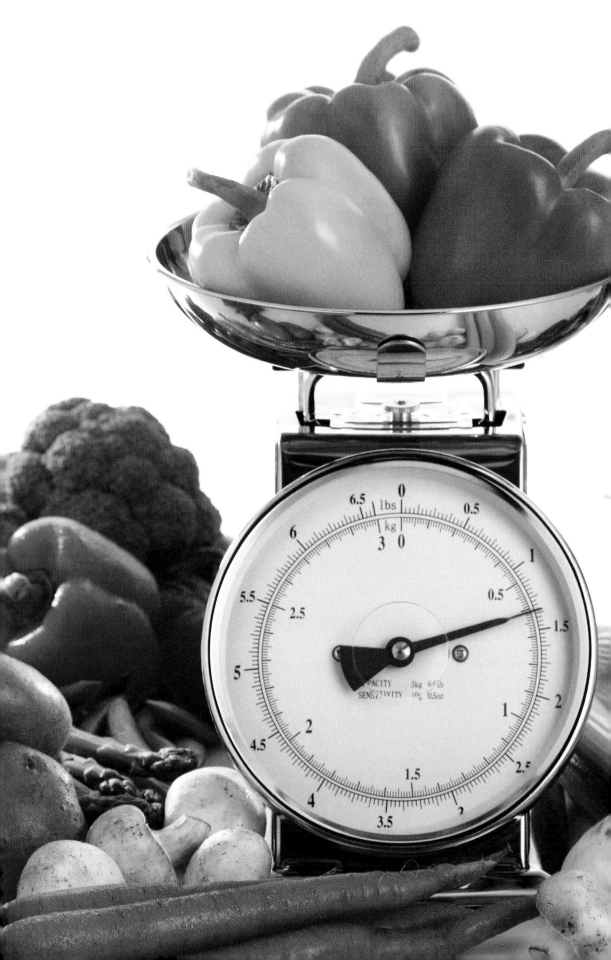

DO NOT CONFORM
ANY LONGER TO THE
PATTERN OF THIS WORLD,
BUT BE TRANSFORMED
BY THE RENEWING OF
YOUR MIND.

- ROMANS 12:2

what's hot, what's not

With so much focus on Best Dressed and Worst Dressed Lists, you'd think someone would have put the same emphasis on what goes *in* our bodies instead of just what goes *on* them. After all, how can you look great on the outside if you don't feel great on the inside?

So, I have created my own version of "What's Hot and What's Not." It's my **Best and Worst Foods** list (just don't expect to see it on the E! Channel any time soon).

1 vegetables

Vegetables are the most nutrient dense of all food groups. They contain mostly fiber and almost no sugar, so they help regulate your blood sugar levels. Veggies are also alkaline in nature, so they will help reduce acidity in your body. So, load up on a wide variety of vegetables.

my favorite veggies:

	Leafy Greens	The most nutrient dense foods. Contain the most vitamins and minerals such as potassium and Vitamin K, as well as xanthein and lutein (antioxidants that fight disease).
	Red Cabbage	Good for your digestive tract. Part of the cruciferous family of veggies (known as the "disease fighters").
	Carrots	Super high in beta carotene, which is great for your eyes.
	Red Bell Peppers	High in vitamin C.
	Cauliflower	Another member of the cruciferous family.

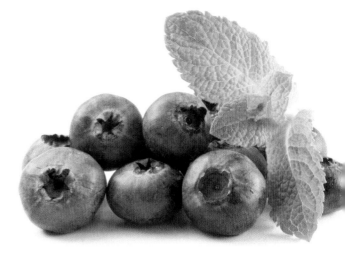

2 fruits

Fruits, especially those of the berry variety, are full of health benefits such as lowering cholesterol and alleviating digestive problems. Not to mention they are nature's sweet desserts! There's nothing better than a fresh strawberry dipped in some dark chocolate fondue. Fruit is also a great mid-afternoon snack to keep your energy levels high.

my favorite fruits:

	Blueberries	Highest in antioxidants. Packed with polyphenols and anthocyanins, which help fight cancer and disease. Great for anti-aging.
	Raspberries	High in fiber, antimicrobial, and a cancer fighter.
	Strawberries	Most nutrient dense fruit. Contains significant levels of phytonutrients and antioxidants.
	Apples	A lot of fiber. Great for your intestines. Helps improve bone density.
	Lemons	Causes your body to be alkaline. Promotes good breath.

3   beans

Humble, inexpensive beans boast big benefits: they can reduce your risk of heart disease and stroke, help prevent cancer, and even save you money. In addition, beans are a good source of B vitamins, potassium, and fiber, which promotes digestive health. As if that isn't enough, they are a great and less expensive source of high quality protein.

my favorite beans:

	Kidney Beans	Good source of fiber. Prevents blood sugar levels from rising too rapidly after a meal (perfect for diabetes).
	Black Beans	Rich in antioxidants with a wide variety of uses. Great fiber source.
	Garbanzo Beans	Source of folic acid, fiber, manganese, and minerals such as iron, copper, zinc, and magnesium.
	Lentils	Very nutrient dense. Source of vitamin C. Shown to reduce risk of heart disease.
	Adzuki Beans	Great source of magnesium, potassium, iron, copper, and B vitamins. Helps reduce blood pressure.

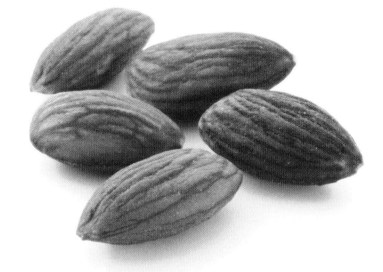

4 nuts + seeds

Nuts are tiny little powerhouses. They contain a host of nutrients that battle heart disease and diabetes, boost brain function and the immune system, and can help you lose weight (Yes, I said *lose* weight).

my favorite nuts:

	Almonds	Anti-inflammatory, high protein source. When used in moderation, helps with weight loss.
	Pecans	Source of oleic acid (which aids in preventing breast cancer). Helps lower bad cholesterol. High in antioxidants.
	Cashews	An energizing food. Helps lower risk of heart disease. Also helps fight depression.
	Pumpkin Seeds	Promotes overall prostate health. Contains L-tryptophan, a compound naturally effective against depression.
	Flax Seeds	Helps lower cholesterol and blood pressure. Helps reduce blood sugar levels. Natural laxative.

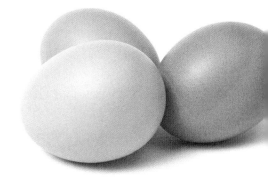

5   organic meats + eggs

There are many health benefits of eating meat; the most obvious is that meat serves as an ideal source of high quality protein. Meat also contains all the essential amino acids that the body requires. The phosphorus content present in meat gets much more easily absorbed than that present in grains. Meat also serves as the main source for the intake of vitamin B12.

Eggs are nature's oval wonders. They are great for the eyes and a good source of choline, which is an important nutrient that helps regulate the brain, nervous system, and cardiovascular system. They are versatile, taste great, and are an easy and quick addition to any meal.

my favorite meat + eggs:

	Wild Salmon	Important source of omega 3 fatty acids, which help reduce inflammation. High in protein. Provides high levels of vitamin D.
	Organic Chicken	More vitamins E, C, and beta-carotene than conventional chicken. Great low-fat source of protein.
	Organic Eggs	Most bio-available protein source (which means your body will be able to use it).
	Grass Fed Beef	High in CLA, which is important to burn fat and lose weight. Also great source of omega 3 fatty acids.
	Venison	High in protein and iron. Low in saturated fat. Good source of B vitamins (for energy and cardio-vascular health).

6   herbs, spices, + gluten-free grains

herbs + spices

In addition to making food taste amazing, herbs and spices have been used for centuries for endless reasons. Their uses range from common ailments to over-all health, weight loss, and more. Herbs can offer the body nutrients it does not always receive, either from a poor diet, or environmental deficiencies in the soil and air. They are great body balancers that help regulate body functions. *And did I mention they taste amazing?*

my favorite herbs:

 Garlic   Great for your complexion. Acts as an anti-viral, anti-bacterial, and anti-parasite. Aids in cleaning arteries.

Cinnamon   Acts as a blood sugar regulator and a potent antioxidant.

Turmeric   Natural anti-inflammatory, great for alleviating joint pain.

Basil   Tastes great! Good source of flavonoids, which help protect cells from damage.

 Ginger   Reduces pain and inflammation. May help fight disease, especially cancer. Helps relieve migraines. Good for nausea.

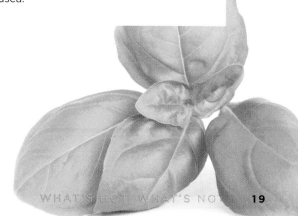

gluten-free grains

While not in my top five real foods, I recommend grains in small and moderate portions—and always non-processed and gluten-free! These types of grains were used thousands of years ago in traditional diets, but modern food processing stepped in and destroyed the goodness of grains. If you have an intolerance or allergy to wheat, as do 1 out of every 133 adults in the United States, then gluten-free and sprouted grains are the way to go.

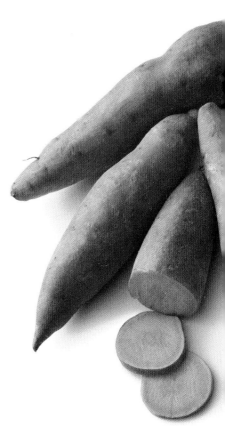

my favorite grains:

	Sweet Potatoes	While it's not a grain, it's still higher in carbohydrates. Rich in Vitamin A and potassium. Good for inflammatory bowel conditions.
	Quinoa	An excellent food for nursing mothers as it stimulates breast milk. Rich in iron, calcium, phosphorus, and B vitamins.
	Brown + Wild Rice	A healthy dose of B vitamins (the highest levels of all grains) and high fiber content. Helps control blood sugar. High in folic acid and niacin.
	Sprouted Gluten-Free Grains (Spelt, Millet)	Still has nutrients intact, easier to digest and lower on the glycemic index than processed grains. Also high in B vitamins.

what's not: five worst fake foods

Now that we've discussed what you should eat, we obviously need to talk about what NOT to eat. There are five major categories of fake foods that you need to avoid at all costs in order to bring healing to your body:

1 refined sugar

Warning! Refined sugar is lethal when ingested by humans!

Think I'm exaggerating? I wish I were. Sugar is not only devoid of any and all nutrients, it's actually worse than "empty"—sugar is an anti-nutrient that drains and leaches the body of precious vitamins and minerals through the demand that sugar's digestion, detoxification, and elimination makes upon your entire system.

Excess sugar affects every organ in the body. Sugar is initially stored in the liver in the form of glucose. Your liver can only handle so much sugar, and excess sugar ends up in your bloodstream damaging your arteries, pancreas, and then eventually gets turned into fat on your belly, butt, and thighs.

Any one left to wonder why obesity is on the rise? It's pretty obvious. We must stop the sugar and switch to one of the many sweet alternatives that I'll discuss in the next section.

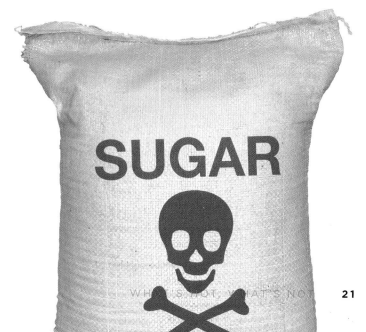

2 hydrogenated oils

When most people think of cooking oils, what immediately comes to mind is vegetable or canola oil. These oils are found in abundance in the grocery stores because they are cheap to produce, due in part to the government subsidization of corn crops. But these oils, along with oils like soybean, cottonseed, and safflower, are highly processed and rancid. I can't encourage you strongly enough to remove them from your diet!

Trans fats are found in partially hydrogenated fats and oils. They are dangerous because they are incorporated into the body's cell membranes and interfere with normal cell metabolism and other chemical reactions. Hydrogenated fats have been linked to a wide array of health dangers such as birth defects, cancer, diabetes, heart disease, learning disabilities, digestive disorders, obesity, sexual dysfunction, skin reactions, increased cholesterol levels, and immune system impairment.

Quite an exhaustive list, wouldn't you agree? How many of us would like to avoid any one of the ills on this list? Well, it's up to you. Avoid hydrogenated oils, and use the many healthy alternatives we'll talk about in the next section.

3 processed grains/white stuff

White bread, white pasta, and white rice have become staples in the Standard American Diet (the SAD Diet). Even though there is a trend toward seemingly healthy wheat bread or whole grain pasta, these grains are still processed and refined—to the point that I would not even call them food.

Carbohydrates are an important part of your diet, but your main source of carbs should be coming from fruits and vegetables rather than refined grains. Refined carbohydrates have been linked to diseases of the heart, kidneys, liver, and pancreas. Refined carbohydrates are connected to allergies, ADHD, anorexia, bone loss, depression, diabetes, Celiac Disease, and gluten intolerance.

Bottom line: Refined carbohydrates are fake foods and should be avoided if you want to build health in your body. Enough Said.

4   pasteurized dairy (aka scary dairy)

Most of us take it for granted that milk and other foods are pasteurized and homogenized. When certain practices go unquestioned, we accept them as being "just the way things are." But pasteurization and homogenization denature foods. They alter the chemical structure of food, make fats rancid, destroy nutrients, and cause the formation of free radicals.

Pasteurization denatures milk in multiple ways. The process destroys vitamin A completely and destroys more than a third of the B vitamins. It also destroys the enzyme phosphatase, which is needed to absorb calcium. So, that just busted the biggest myth of all—that milk builds healthy bones. Protein, fat, and sugar particles in denatured milk easily pass through the intestinal lining and cause inflammation and allergic reactions.

It's not just dairy anymore either. Pasteurization is used on everything from fruit juices to shelled nuts. Every day, more foods are pasteurized to make up for unsanitary conditions, destroying the natural bacteria and enzymes that would normally counteract the growth of pathogens. Homogenized products have been linked to rising rates of cancer and heart disease.

Pasteurization is not a natural process that our food was meant to undergo. So do yourself and your kids a favor and make the switch to one of the dairy alternatives that we'll discuss a little later.

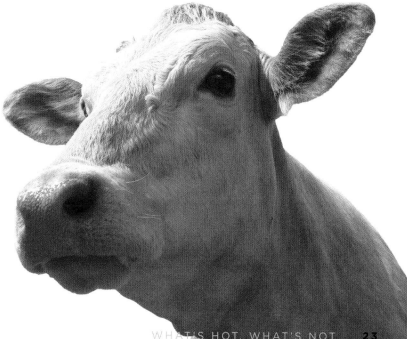

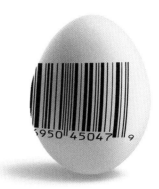

5 conventional meats + eggs

Let's take a pound of nice, fresh meat and add in some nitrates, hormones, and antibiotics. Yep, believe it or not, it's possible to turn meat into a fake food. And folks, the saying is true: You are what you eat. And when it comes to conventionally grown livestock, it's more like:

You are what you eat . . . what they ate.

The terms "non-organic" and "conventional" meats and eggs usually refer to the fact that the animals may have been fed antibiotics, hormones, ground up remains of other animals, and other dangerous substances that often end up in these foods fed to us. The growing use of chemicals is primarily used for the purpose of fattening up the animals quickly for slaughter, and their use is a disaster for the health of the animals and, of course, the humans who eat them.

Conventional meat and poultry are fed conventional foods, and more specifically, grains. Why? Carbohydrates are just as effective at fattening animals as humans. The pesticides, herbicides, fungicides, and fertilizers in the grain are then stored as toxins in the fat of the animals.

Because conventionally raised animals are kept in confined quarters 24/7, they do not get the exercise they need to stay healthy. Between the poor quality of food and the close quarters, sickness spreads like wildfire through the herds and barns. Consequently, antibiotics are used on an ongoing basis in an attempt to keep the animals alive—and as a result, we ingest the antibiotics when we eat the sick animals. It's a vicious and dangerous cycle.

One common complaint is the price of organic meat; and yes, it is often higher than conventional meat. I have two pieces of advice to offer on this front: 1. Watch for specials at your local health food grocery store and 2. Spend less money on something else that is a lower priority and buy organic meat!

6   artificial sweeteners

The idea that sugar substitutes are healthy alternatives is rooted in the American mindset. However, this couldn't be any more untrue. Worse yet, the prevalence of artificial sweeteners, corn syrup, and refined sugars in the majority of American foods has created a country of sweet-addicts.

Due to the extravagant amount of sweeteners in the majority of our foods, many of us can no longer detect natural sweetness in healthy plant foods. We're not made to handle this extreme amount of sweetness. This excess triggers unhealthy food cravings and addiction, and when we take in these low-nutrient foods and drinks, we have less room for nutritious food.

Are you one of the millions of Americans who think that you are somehow avoiding the weight gain associated with soda by drinking the diet versions? Think again! Diet sodas and sweetened water beverages are actually linked to weight gain! Artificial sweeteners are bad news.

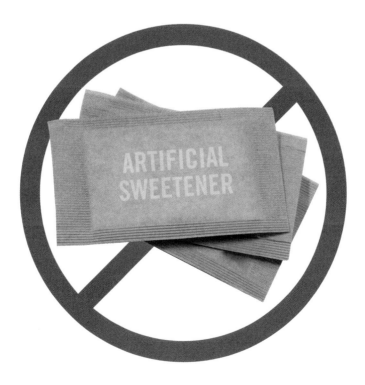

Let's take a look at the most common artificial sweeteners and why we should avoid them:

aspartame
(EQUAL, NUTRASWEET, FOUND IN MANY DIET SODA BRANDS)

Aspartame is 180 times sweeter than sugar. The FDA file of complaints concerning aspartame ingestion includes reports of dizziness, headaches, and memory loss. Some studies suggest it is a carcinogen (yes, that means cancer causing).

saccharin
(SWEET N' LOW, FOUND IN MANY PROCESSED FOODS, DIABETIC PRODUCTS)

Saccharin is 300 times sweeter than sugar. The public stopped purchasing products made with the sweetener when they learned of its possible link to cancer. However, studies didn't decisively prove this link, so it is once again common in many artificially sweetened foods. Saccharin is linked, however, to sweetness addiction, obesity, and overeating.

sucralose
(SPLENDA, COMMON IN SUGARFREE BAKED GOODS, BREADS, FRUIT JUICES)

Sucralose is 600 times sweeter than table sugar. Sucralose was an accidental discovery; it was originally part of a new insecticide compound. But Splenda is "made from sugar" right?

First of all, why is that a good thing? Sugar is toxic! Secondly, the nutrients that many sweetened waters are said to contain are often present in only the most miniscule amounts or are in forms that our bodies can't make use of. Chlorinated compounds (classified as carcinogens) such as sucralose were thought to pass through the body undigested. Recent research has found that up to forty percent of chlorinated compounds become stockpiled in the intestinal tract, kidneys, and liver.

We can reverse our addiction to unhealthy sweeteners and restore our ability to taste the natural sweetness in whole foods over time. It will seem difficult at first, but I can't encourage you strongly enough to put down the diet sodas and the colored sweetener packets! These chemicals are foreign to our bodies and will not help you achieve any of your health goals.

the abc's of cooking, equipment, and label reading

Everything we need to know, we learned in kindergarten?? I don't know about your kindergarten class, but we had nothing but juice boxes and cookies lying around. If we all ate like that for the rest of our lives, there'd be a lot fewer of us. And for that matter, Mrs. Richards never taught me how to do my taxes. So, I guess there are some things to learn beyond age five. In this section, you will find a few crash courses in some of the basics of healthy eating—you know, stuff you may not have learned in between naptime and recess.

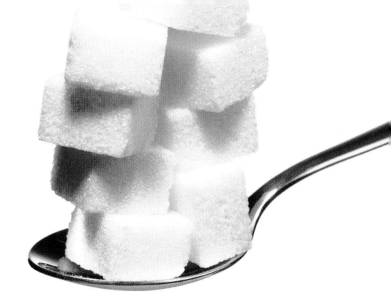

sugar 101

so, no sugar? no artificial sugar?
what about my sweet tooth? it has demands!

Well, there's good news. There are several alternative sweeteners that are natural and even sweeter than sugar in some cases. These sugars aren't full of dangerous chemicals and won't affect your blood sugar as much as processed sugars. But they should still be used in very small amounts. Sugar in large amounts is toxic to the body. Here is my list of the best sweeteners. They are listed in the order in which I recommend them:

stevia

Stevia is my top choice for natural sweetener. Packing an incredibly sweet punch, stevia has many health properties. The body does not metabolize the sweet glycosides from the stevia leaf, so there is no caloric intake. And perhaps best of all, stevia doesn't adversely affect blood glucose levels and may be used freely by diabetics.

xylitol

Pure xylitol is a white crystalline substance that looks and tastes like sugar. Xylitol is a safe, natural sweetener that's also good for your teeth, stabilizes insulin and hormone levels, and promotes good health. It has the same sweetness as sugar but with 40 percent fewer calories and without the insulin releasing effects of sugar.

raw honey

Raw honey aids in digestive health. Honey does not ferment in the stomach because it is easily absorbed and there is no danger of a bacterial invasion. Honey may also help with allergies, infections, and arthritis.

coconut nectar

Coconut nectar is the sap that comes from coconut blossoms. It is extremely low on the Glycemic scale, and it also contains 17 amino acids, minerals, vitamin C, and broad-spectrum B vitamins. Not to mention it has a nearly neutral pH.

maple syrup

Maple syrup has been shown to promote heart health. The zinc supplied by maple syrup, in addition to acting as an antioxidant, has other functions that can decrease the progression of atherosclerosis.

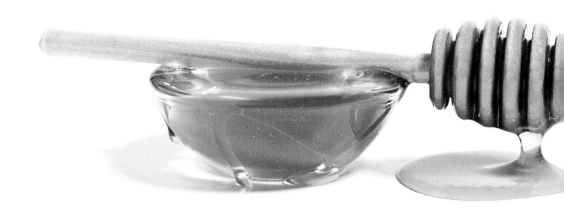

Once you make the switch to alternative sugars, you can still make your favorite desserts and other meals that require refined sugar. All you have to do is substitute in the good stuff for the bad stuff. In order to make sure your food comes out tasting right, I have included conversion charts for using stevia in place of sugar in recipes.

Remember, stevia is far sweeter than sugar, so be sure to use the conversion chart when substituting in a recipe. (Note: No conversion chart is needed for xylitol. Spoon for spoon, you can measure it just like sugar).

Long live your sweet tooth—in moderation, of course!!

NOTE: *Apart from stevia, all other sugar alternatives should be eaten in small amounts and used sparingly.*

equivalents chart
for sugar substitution with stevia

Sugar	Stevia Powder
2 tsp	1/2 tsp
1/4 cup	3 tsp
1/2 cup	6 tsp
1 cup	12 tsp

Sugar	Stevia Liquid
2 tsp	1/4 tsp
1/4 cup	1/2 tsp

fats + oils 101

Now that we've discussed hydrogenated oils among the Five Worst Fake Foods, let's talk about the healthy alternatives. The good news? Once you switch to these healthy oils, you won't even miss the processed, bad fats. In fact, you'll prefer the good oils because they will make your food taste even better. Here are the oils and fats I recommend for cooking:

coconut oil
USED FOR COOKING AT MEDIUM TO MEDIUM-HIGH HEAT

The coconut has gotten a bad rap over the years because of one reason: Saturated fat has gotten a bad rap. Because of this, most have shied away from using anything related to the coconut due to the fact that the fat content in coconuts is composed of 98 percent saturated fat. But as I am sure you are aware of by now, there are good fats and there are bad fats.

Is all saturated fat bad? No. So, what makes coconut oil's fat different from the other oils, especially other saturated fats? The difference is in the fat molecules themselves. All fats are composed of molecules called fatty acids. There are two classifications of fatty acids: 1. Saturation level, and 2. Length of the carbon chain within each fat molecule. Most of us know about the saturation classification, so let's discuss the second one.

There are three lengths: Short-chain fatty acids (SCFA), medium-chain fatty acids (MCFA), and long-chain fatty acids (LCFA). Coconut oil is composed predominately of medium-chain fatty acids (MCFA). MCFA are proven to help burn fat and lose weight. In fact, it is the same kind of fat found in breast milk.

Researchers have found that these fatty acids may prove useful in combating antibiotic-resistant bacteria and viruses. So, it is the presence of the MCFA like lauric acid in coconut oil that makes it so healthy and my number one pick for cooking.

grapeseed oil

Grapeseed oil is a light, sweet and nutty, flavored oil extracted from the seeds of different varieties of grapes. Grapes have been known for their medicinal and nutritive properties for thousands of years. Grapeseed oil may help lower cholesterol, especially the harmful LDL cholesterol. It has also been found to increase HDL, the good cholesterol, which reduces risk of heart disease.

Certain compounds found in grapeseed oil have been linked to improved vision, increased flexibility of joints, and better blood circulation. This oil can also be effective in reducing the symptoms associated with allergies and asthma, as it suppresses the production of histamine (an amine released by the immune system during allergic reactions).

Use grapeseed oil for baking, frying, salad dressings, marinades, and sauces.

sesame oil

USED FOR COOKING AT MEDIUM TO MEDIUM-HIGH HEAT

Another one of my favorites is sesame oil, though I don't use it as much as coconut and grapeseed oil. Unlike olive oil, sesame oil does not easily oxidize when it is heated. Sesame oil is very high in linoleic acid, one of the two essential fatty acids (EFAs) our bodies cannot produce but have to get from outside sources. Essential fatty acids are necessary for normal growth and for healthy blood, arteries, and nerves. They keep the skin and other tissues youthful and healthy by preventing dryness.

Since the explosive growth of food processing, particularly oil and grain refinement, EFA deficiencies and imbalances are becoming more common. Linoleic acid deficiencies include hair loss, skin eruptions, mood swings, arthritis, infections, and even heart, liver, and kidney disease.

Sesame oil is a great way to supplement your body with this essential fatty acid.

olive oil

Most of us have heard over the years that olive oil is one of the best oils to use. But that's not entirely true, and here's why: though it's a good fat, you don't want to cook with it. Olive oil turns into a bad fat above medium heat (anything above 200-250 degrees, which isn't all that hot when it comes to cooking). When you first pour olive oil into a pan, it's green and fresh. But have you ever seen that smoke coming off the pan after letting the olive oil heat for a few minutes? As the temperature rises above 250 degrees, all the nutrients are literally burned out of the oil, and you are left with black, toxic fumes.

If you love your Extra Virgin Olive Oil, use it in your salad dressings, but don't cook with it when there are so many other better alternatives.

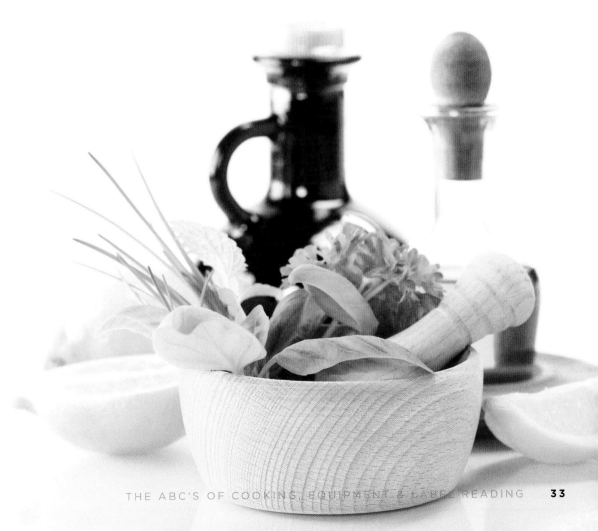

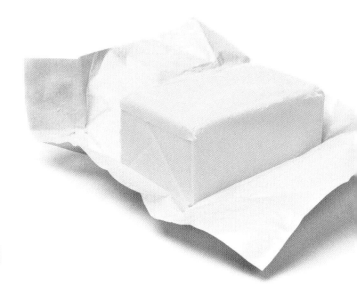

dairy + milk 101

Now that I've told you to steer clear of dairy, it may seem like all hope is lost, and you might as well close down your kitchen altogether and never step foot into another restaurant. The average American has at least one serving of something dairy every day, and more like four servings. We are a dairy-driven nation. But do not despair. As always, I am here to provide you with some healthy alternatives to conventional dairy products.

organic butter

Not all dairy products are bad for you. In fact, one of the healthiest whole foods you can include in your diet is butter. Hard to believe, right? Well believe it! Butter is truly better than margarine or other vegetable spreads.

Despite unjustified warnings about saturated fat from well-meaning, albeit misinformed, experts, the list of butter's benefits is impressive: Butter is full of vitamins, minerals, and MCFA that greatly benefit overall health as we saw in the section on coconut oil. Butter also contains conjugated linoleic acid (CLA), which is a natural fat burner.

When looking for quality butter, raw and cultured is best. However, depending on where you live, this might be hard to find. Organic butter is your next best thing, with store bought butter being the last option (because that butter is made from conventionally raised cows and all the chemicals that come with them).

It's worth a few extra cents to get high quality butter for you and your family.

coconut milk

Coconut milk is one of my favorite things to use when cooking Asian curry dishes or making smoothies. My kitchen is always stocked with a carton. I also use it as an alternative to pasteurized dairy in recipes that call for milk. Coconut milk is made from crushing and squeezing the meat of coconuts. It has a similar consistency to milk without all the added hormones, chemicals, and health problems. You may not start out drinking it straight from the carton or can, but coconut milk is a healthy and delicious alternative to cow's milk.

other non-dairy milks

There are a variety of other non-dairy or vegan choices out there when it comes to milk.

Hemp milk is one popular choice, with a rich, sweet taste and full of amino acids, vitamin A, magnesium, phosphorus, zinc, iron, and lots of calcium. Other milk options include almond milk, which has a predictably nutty taste, and rice milk, a light alternative to dairy or soy.

While my top pick goes to coconut milk, experiment with these other milks for picky kids or for your own choosy taste buds.

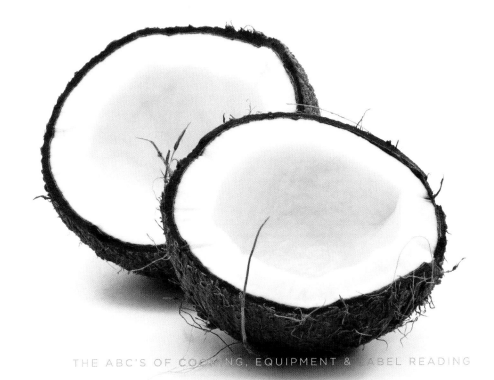

a word about soy

Why didn't I mention soymilk? Well, there are a few reasons, but I will give you the Cliff's Notes version. Soymilk contains phytoestrogens, which are chemicals that affect the body in the same way that the female hormone estrogen does. This is said to negatively affect people who regularly consume soy, causing problems with their thyroids and possibly even fertility.

Studies also show the possibility of a rise in the risk for endometrial cancers when women consume high levels of phytoestrogens. And even more disturbing, babies who are fed soy formula are essentially fed the equivalents of ten birth control pills.

While fermented soy products are safer to consume, the jury is still out on soy products as a whole. There is a lot of evidence out there that proves the vast majority of soy is genetically modified with aluminum added in. It's safe to say there is enough research out there to suggest that you might want to take a second look at soymilk before buying it.

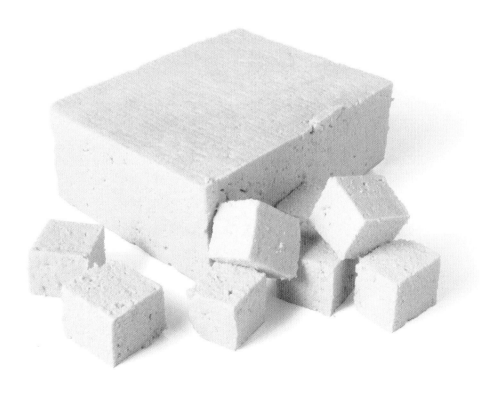

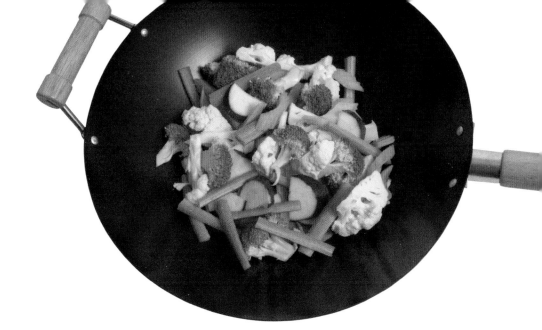

cooking 101

Once the oils are heating, and you're ready to fire up some veggies, we need to discuss how you should cook them. There are a few rules to live by. Actually, there is really just one rule, and here it is:

The Cooking Rule: Don't overcook!

Here is my preferred order of cooking methods for vegetables and other natural foods (this list does not apply to uncooked meat):

1. Raw
2. Lightly Steam
3. Sauté (stirfry)
4. Baked

When preparing meat, just use some common sense. Lightly baking or pan-frying meat in a healthy oil such as coconut oil is better than deep-frying, and it is always better than using a microwave.

It's really very basic. The longer you cook, the more nutrients get burned off or destroyed. Why bother switching to organic veggies or organic meats if you're just going to suck everything good out of them all by using improper cooking methods?

label reading 101

We've all heard that the best place to stay in a grocery store is around the perimeter—or in other words, the items that require refrigeration (likely because they are not laden with preservatives before being stuffed into a can or box). Well, of course I agree with this familiar grocery store rule. But let's be honest. Sometimes we need the aisle stuff! It's practically impossible not to step into an aisle now and then. So what do we do once we venture into the forbidden middle aisles?

We read labels. There are literally hundreds of chemicals used in food that most Americans eat every day. But luckily, there are five main ingredients that the vast majority of processed food manufacturers use. So those are the ones we are going to learn and watch out for. Listed below are the Top Five Villains of Processed Food and some of their aliases.

the five villains of processed food

Hydrogenated Oils	You will see these listed in a wide array of oils such as corn, soybean, cottonseed, vegetable, and canola.
Food Additives	There are tons of them, but the most common additives are yellow 5 and monosodium glutamate.
Sugar	Look for ingredients like corn syrup, high fructose corn syrup, sugar, and dextrose.
Artificial Sweeteners	This could be listed as any of the chemical laden sweeteners. Look for the big three: Sucralose (Splenda), Aspartame, and Saccharin.
White or Wheat Flour	The presence of wheat (commonly the number one or two ingredient) means that this food has been heavily over processed. Usually accompanied by the word "enriched."

Yes, label reading is important. Yes, you need to learn how to spot the five big villains of the grocery aisles and avoid them. But in general, there's really just one rule to follow. And ironically, it's a simple one: Simple is better. The fewer ingredients, the healthier it probably is. If you are reading an ingredient label and need to pause for some water or a nap in the middle, that's too many ingredients. The goal is to keep our foods as close to the way nature made them as possible.

pesticides: to buy or not to buy organic

Label reading is the first step toward putting healthy, real food in our bodies. But what about all those fruits, veggies, and meats that don't come with a handy label?

One question I always get is, *how important is it to buy organic foods versus non organic?* The answer is it can be very important depending on the food you're eating. The word "organic" typically means that something has not been sprayed with pesticides and other dangerous chemicals. Faker than fake, pesticides are definitely NOT real food, not to mention the fact that they've been linked to ADHD and other neurological health problems.

In order to help you decide when it's safe to buy conventionally and when it's better to go organic, there are certain foods that I strongly urge you to buy organic. At the top of the list are meat and dairy products. And to help you decide what conventional produce to avoid, here is a list of the 12 foods that are most contaminated with pesticides:

the tainted twelve

Peaches	Nectarines	Lettuce
Apples	Strawberries	Imported Grapes
Bell Peppers	Cherries	Carrots
Celery	Kale	Pears

Other foods are not sprayed as often or have thick skin to protect the food. Here is a list of the sixteen least contaminated foods that are okay to buy conventional when you can't afford to buy organic:

the safe sixteen

Onions	Broccoli	Kiwi
Sweet corn	Tomatoes	Papayas
Asparagus	Sweet potatoes	Watermelon
Sweet peas	Avocadoes	Grapefruit
Cabbage	Pineapples	
Eggplant	Mangoes	

By following these tables and avoiding the most heavily pesticide-ridden foods, you can greatly reduce your pesticide exposure!

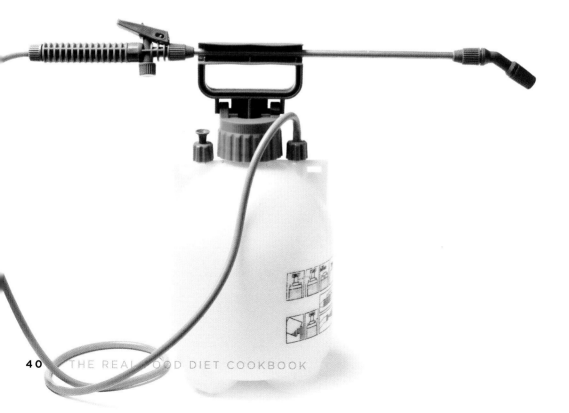

equipment 101

Okay, we're doing pretty well so far. We know what fake foods to avoid and what real foods will transform our health. But honestly, that is all a bit pointless if you close this book and start cooking with the wrong equipment. Remember the whole point of eating real food is to limit the exposure of chemicals and additives to your body and replace them with lifegiving nutrients. Well, shockingly, many of your kitchen's most used items are filled with as many toxins, if not more, as the fake foods. So, let's have a quick lesson in what to throw away, and then as always, I'll tell you what equipment to keep.

throw this stuff away

nonstick and teflon cookware

Non-stick or Teflon pans have a coating applied to them that prevents food from sticking and makes cleaning up easier. That's super! But at what cost do we demand this easy cleanup? At a great cost. Teflon pans are linked to the following health problems:

- Childhood development problems and diseases
- Liver, pancreas, testicular, and mammary gland diseases
- Growth of tumors
- Disrupted thyroid hormones

It is predicted that in the next few years, Teflon will be banned. I guess the truth is finally getting out about these chemically laden, disease-causing pans. To make matters worse, Teflon pans are involved in one or more class action lawsuits at any given time. Is that the type of product you want to use to fix food for your family?

microwaves

Microwaves alter the very chemical structure of food. As a consequence, the human body cannot metabolize the unknown by-products created in micro-waved food. They also destroy the minerals, vitamins, and nutrients of even the healthiest foods.

Adding to the list of dangers, continual use of microwaves greatly alters or even shuts down both male and female hormone production. To add insult to injury, vegetables, which are by their very natures diseases fighters, are changed into cancerous free radicals when cooked in microwaves. Get those things out of your home (even if it does match your stove and fridge). Or just use it for extra kitchen storage.

Switching to a convection oven or just using your stovetop is a great alternative to using a microwave.

plastic containers

Plastic is not universally "bad" in the kitchen. Plastic can have its uses when it comes to storing something in the fridge (plastic bags for veggies, for instance). And we can't do much about the fact that many foods come in plastic. So, plastic has its place, but that place is not cooking or heating.

Store food in glass when you can, and try to avoid plastic due to the fact that it contains BPAs and pthalates, which disrupt your endocrine system. But if you do use it, make sure you don't heat it up.

stainless steel, cast iron, and ceramic cookware

Alternative metal and ceramic cookware is perfect for the healthy chef. Because the surface of these pots and pans can't get scratched and chipped like Teflon, they have fewer cracks to harbor dirt, grime, or bacteria. This cookware is great for cooks who swear by Teflon for its ease of care because metal and ceramic pots and pans are just as easy to care for—and maybe even easier!

And the added bonus is that they stay attractive longer and require minimal care, since they won't chip or easily rust. With proper care, alternative cookware has a useful life expectancy of over 100 years. Yes, our pans may outlive us.

high quality blender

Many of the recipes in this cookbook will require you to mix and blend ingredients. For this reason, every kitchen should be equipped with a top-notch blender. In my experience, all blenders are not created equal. You get what you pay for with a blender, so invest in a good one.

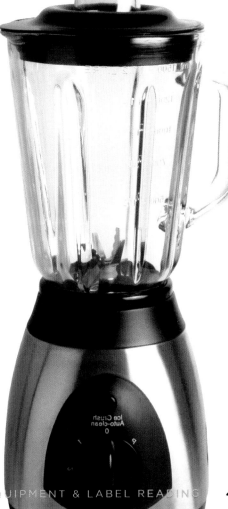
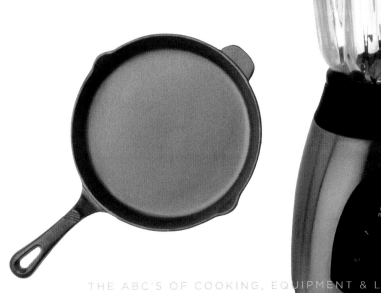

WHEN YOU FIND
YOURSELF ON THE SIDE
OF THE MAJORITY, IT'S TIME
TO PAUSE AND REFLECT.

- MARK TWAIN

less that/ more this

I have a complaint to lodge against modern diet plans. It's that they all seem to have one annoying thing in common: forbidden food lists that make you feel like you are going to have to sacrifice everything in life if you want to lose weight and be healthy. So, they take away all of life's pleasures, and leave us with big, hungry, empty stomachs.

I say if you were going to remove something from your diet, it'd be nice to have a replacement in mind. That's what I've done throughout the previous sections. So, in an attempt to keep you from feeling deprived, hopeless, and hungry, I've provided you with a short list of replacement foods for some of your favorite meals and snacks.

On the tables in this section, you will see a value for Glycemic Load. So, I'd like to take a moment to explain the significance of this number and how you can use it to choose healthy foods.

glycemic load

The Glycemic Index is a measure of how quickly carbohydrates are digested. The GI was created to make people aware of how fast foods turn into sugar. For instance, straight sugar is the highest with a score of 100, white bread 96, wheat bread 75, oatmeal 50, apple 35, and veggies 0-10.

Typically the lower the score the better. But not in all cases. For instance, the glycemic index of a carrot is 70, but it has very few carbs. So it really doesn't have much of an effect on your blood sugar. Oatmeal on the other hand, though it has a better index rating at 50 points, has about 6 times the amount of carbohydrates, making the true effect on blood sugar much greater.

Glycemic Load measures the carbohydrate content and the glycemic index of food to give an idea of the blood-sugar-raising potential of carbohydrates. The Glycemic Load is the most practical way to apply the Glycemic Index to dieting, and is easily calculated by multiplying a food's Glycemic Index (as a percentage) by the number of net carbohydrates in a given serving. Glycemic Load gives a relative indication of how much that serving of food is likely to increase your blood-sugar levels.

If you are trying to lose weight, monitoring your daily Glycemic Load and keeping it as low as possible should be a primary focus. As a rule of thumb, most nutritional experts consider Glycemic Loads below 10 to be "low," and Glycemic Loads above 20 to be "high." Because Glycemic Load is related to the food's effect on blood sugar, low Glycemic Load meals are often recommended for diabetic control and weight loss.

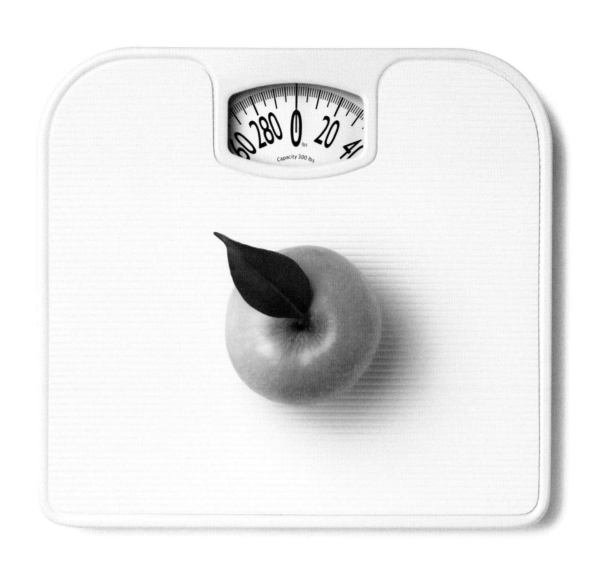

GL = GI/100 × Net Carbs*

(*Net Carbs are equal to the Total Carbohydrates
minus Dietary Fiber)

breakfast

	Less That	More This
Name	Cereal and Milk	Berry Smoothie
Description	Oat or wheat flakes, slightly sweetened, with 2% milk	Blended mix of coconut milk, protein, berries, cinnamon, and stevia
Serving Size	1 1/4 cup cereal, 1 cup milk	1 cup berries, 2 eggs, 1/2 cup coconut milk, cinnamon
Calories	333	330
GLYCEMIC LOAD	38	7
Name	Doughnut	Ezekiel Bread with organic butter
Description	Small glazed doughnut	Sprouted Grains, toasted and spread with organic butter
Serving Size	2 small doughnuts	Large slice with 1 tbsp butter
Calories	400	220
GLYCEMIC LOAD	24	9

lunch

	Less That	More This
Name	Sub Sandwich with Chips	Salad with Grilled Chicken
Description	Cold cut sub with toppings, cheese, and mayo, bag of chips	Fresh Greens, chopped veggies, natural salad dressing (oil & vinegar), grilled chicken
Serving Size	6 inch sub, 10 oz chips	Large salad with 6 oz grilled chicken
Calories	680	360
GLYCEMIC LOAD	33	0

	Less That	More This
Name	Tacos with Chips and Rice	Chicken Salad with side of fresh greens
Description	Beef and Chicken tacos w/ cheese, sour cream, and salsa with a side of tortilla chips and Mexican rice	Grilled chicken, walnuts, grapes, celery, Vegenaise, seasoning
Serving Size	1 beef taco, 1 chicken taco, 10 oz chips, small rice	One large scoop of chicken salad with a large bowl of greens
Calories	640	480
GLYCEMIC LOAD	39	5

snacks

	Less That	More This
Name	Candy Bar	Cherry Snack Bar
Description	Snickers	Dried cherries, nuts, dates
Serving Size	1 bar (4oz)	1 bar (4oz)
Calories	528	200
GLYCEMIC LOAD	41	18
Name	Corn Chips	Gluten Free Rice Crackers
Description	Traditional corn chips such as Fritos made with partially hydrogenated soybean oil	Made with organic brown rice flour, flax seeds, sea salt
Serving Size	25 chips	13 crackers
Calories	160	140
GLYCEMIC LOAD	9	3

dinner

	Less That	More This
Name	Pizza	Pizza
Description	Enriched flour crust, tomato based processed sauce, cheese, pepperoni, sausage	Rice tortilla, sauce, topped with veggies
Serving Size	2 slices	2 slices
Calories	510	290
GLYCEMIC LOAD	28	10
Name	Fried Chicken with Mashed Potatoes	Chicken Tenders and Faux-tatoes
Description	Fried chicken and buttery mashed potatoes	Chicken, gluten-free flour, cauliflower, butter
Serving Size	1 breast, 1 leg, 1 thigh with 8 oz mashed potatoes w/ gravy	3 chicken tenders and a large scoop of faux-tatoes
Calories	820	490
GLYCEMIC LOAD	27	5

dessert

	Less That	More This
Name	Chocolate Milkshake	Chocolate Milkshake
Description	Ice cream and oil based milkshake w/ artificially flavored chocolate and white sugar	Coconut milk, unsweetened cocoa powder, stevia extract, ice
Serving Size	1 medium milkshake	1 large milkshake
Calories	560	230
GLYCEMIC LOAD	37	0
Name	Cheesecake	Raw Cheesecake
Description	Traditional cheesecake made with cream cheese, refined sugar, eggs	Cashews and dates
Serving Size	1 medium slice	1 medium slice
Calories	310	250
GLYCEMIC LOAD	11	0

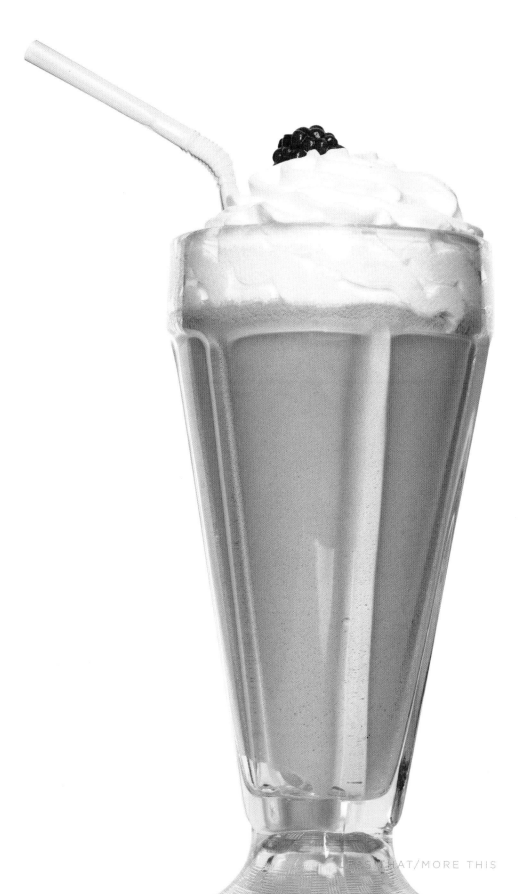

glycemic index

Glucose	Cornflakes	Lifesavers	Rice cakes	Table sugar - sucrose
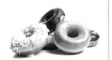				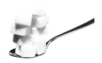
97	84	70	82	65
97	77	68	67	65

Cheerios cereal	Grapenuts cereal	Granola	Bagel	White bread
		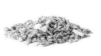		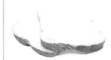
74	67	61	72	70
54	54	40	38	35

All Bran cereal	Whole wheat bread	White rice	Fructose	Baked potato
	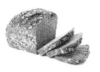			
42	69	72	23	85
33	32	24	23	20

vs. glycemic load

	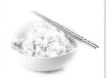		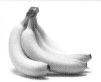	
Oatmeal	**Boiled brown rice**	**Boiled sweet potato**	**Banana**	**Pineapple**
55	55	54	83	66
17	13	13	12	8

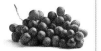		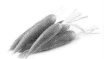		
Grapes	**Beans**	**Carrots**	**Kiwi fruit**	**Apple**
43	30	71	52	39
8	8	7	7	6

		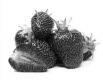		
Orange	**Cherries**	**Strawberries**	**Broccoli**	**Spinach**
43	22	32	25	15
5	4	3	1	0

IN ORDER TO LIVE LIKE NO
ONE ELSE, YOU HAVE TO
LIVE LIKE NO ONE ELSE.

- DAVE RAMSEY

food matching guide

There are countless amounts of guides out there telling us what's best to fix for a baby shower, good ideas for a dinner party, or the best snacks for the big game; but what about what to fix when you're feeling sick and need a boost, need some fuel after a workout, or need to prepare food for fickle kids?

Not sure what to eat?

Well, not anymore. On the next page is a list of categories that you will find marked throughout the recipes. When you see one of these symbols, it means that it has all the best nutrients for what you are facing. So find the category that best suits you, and use its symbol to find all the recipes that fit that category.

AIN'T NOTHING LIKE THE REAL THING BABY...

- MARVIN GAYE

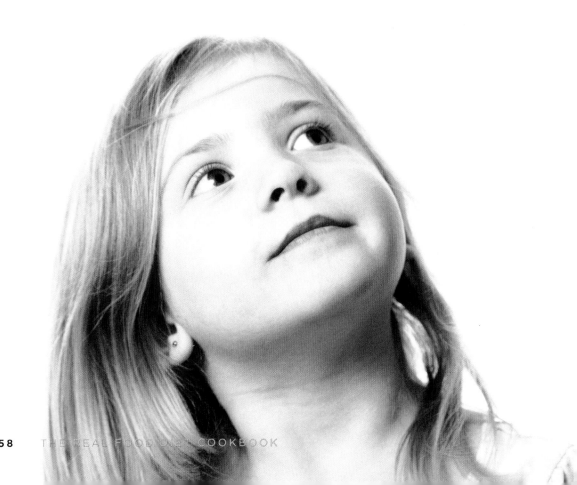

food matching guide

 Quick Recipes Recipes with this symbol can be prepared in less than 30 minutes—and sometimes much faster.

 Raw Foods Recipes These recipes do not require cooking. They are simply foods that are closest to nature, the way food was meant to be. For a quick boost or to jump start weight loss, try these.

 Kids' Favorites Kids can be our toughest critics and definitely our pickiest mouths to please. Recipes with this symbol mean the recipe is kid tested and kid approved!

 Feeling Sick When we feel sick, we immediately think of chicken soup. But chicken soup (the processed kind) can actually do more harm than good. Next time you're feeling under the weather, try these recipes instead.

 Low Energy/ Working Late Our lives are constantly moving forward, and sometimes it's hard to keep up. Recipes with this symbol are filled with ingredients such as cinnamon that can help naturally increase energy levels and give you a boost.

 Post Workout It's hard to know exactly what to eat after a hard workout. These recipes are perfect for a post workout pick-me-up and refresher.

 Inflammation (Arthritis) Pain Inflammation and arthritis pain can be greatly reduced by eating the right foods. The recipes are especially high in ingredients like curry, turmeric, and nuts like almonds.

breakfast

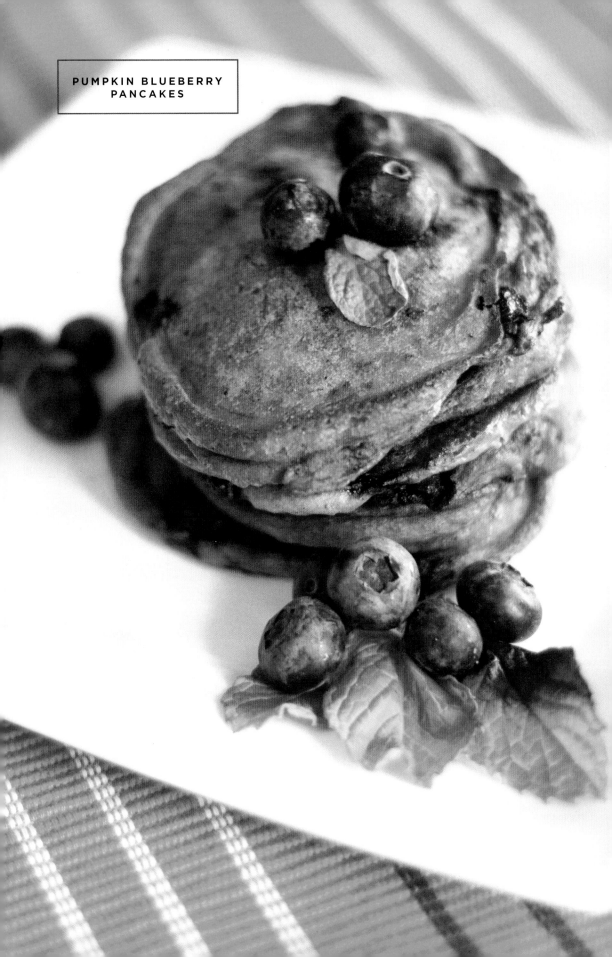

PUMPKIN BLUEBERRY
PANCAKES

Pumpkin Blueberry Pancakes

1 c. gluten-free pancake mix

2 eggs

1/2 c. coconut milk

1/2 c. canned pumpkin

1/2 c. fresh or frozen blueberries

1 tsp. vanilla

1 tsp. cinnamon

2 Tbsp. butter

> Mix all ingredients (through cinnamon) together in a bowl.

> Heat butter in a large skillet over medium heat and drop a scant 1/4 cup of batter into pan. Cook, flipping once, until golden on each side.

Breakfast Berry Smoothie

1/2 cup coconut milk

1 scoop protein powder or 2 eggs

1 c. frozen berries

1/2 tsp. cinnamon

stevia to taste

> Place all ingredients in a blender and blend until frothy.

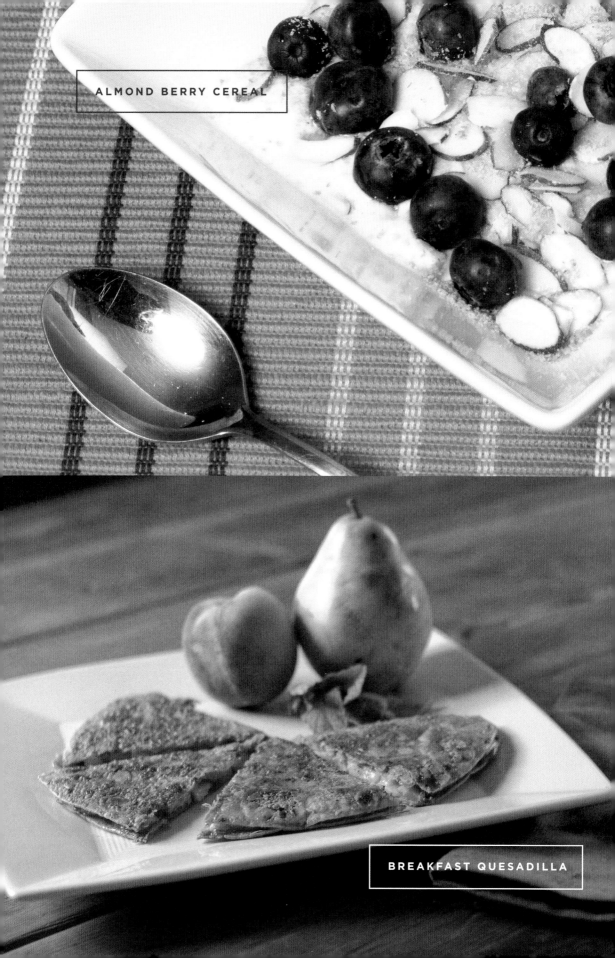

ALMOND BERRY CEREAL

BREAKFAST QUESADILLA

Almond Berry Cereal

4 Tbsp. sliced almonds

4 Tbsp. flax meal

1/2 c. blueberries

1 tsp. cinnamon

4 Tbsp. coconut milk

> Place almonds, coconut milk, flax meal, and blueberries in a bowl.

> Sprinkle with cinnamon.

Breakfast Quesadilla

1 peach, peeled
& diced `

1 pear, peeled
& diced

1/4 c. almond butter

cinnamon to taste

1 Tbsp. coconut oil
or organic butter

1 Tbsp. honey

4 brown rice tortillas

> On the center of the tortilla, spread almond butter and top it with the diced peaches and pears. Drizzle the fruit with honey and sprinkle cinnamon on top. Place a second tortilla on top.

> In a large skillet over medium heat, melt coconut oil or butter.

> Place quesadilla in the skillet, flipping once, until both sides are golden brown and crispy. Repeat with remaining tortillas.

> Drizzle with honey and serve.

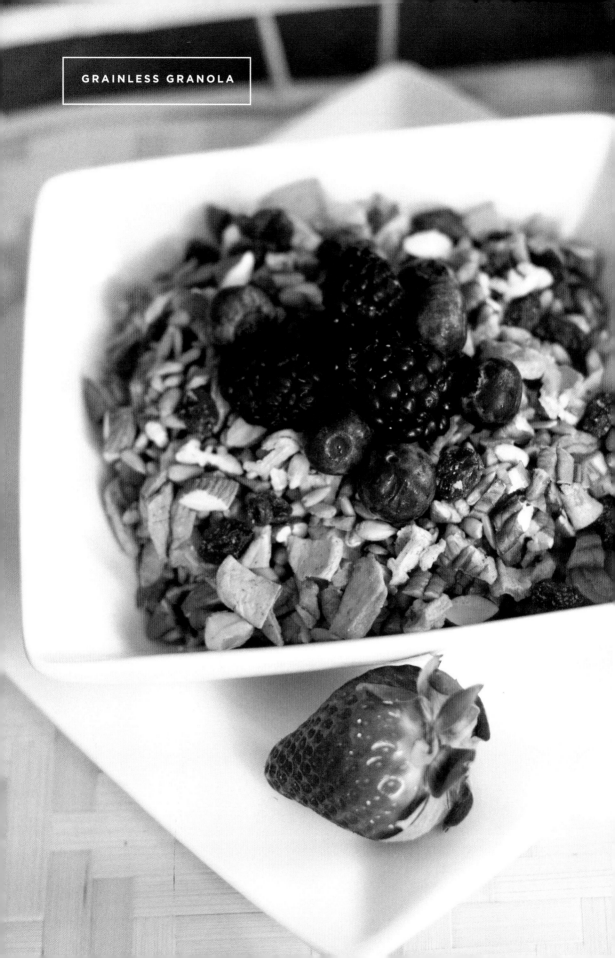

Grainless Granola

1 c. chopped raw pecans or walnuts

1 c. chopped dried apples

1 c. raisins

1 c. raw sunflower seeds

1/2 c. chopped raw almonds

pinch of ground cloves, cinnamon & nutmeg

> Toss all ingredients together in a large bowl.

> Serve by itself or with coconut or almond milk and blueberries.

Turkey Breakfast Sausage

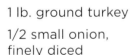

1 lb. ground turkey

1/2 small onion, finely diced

1/4 tsp. each: cumin, marjoram, black pepper, oregano, cayenne pepper, ginger

1/2. tsp. each: dried basil, thyme, sage

2 tsp. sea salt

2 Tbsp. Mary's Gone Crackers, crushed

1 egg, lightly beaten

2 Tbsp. raw or organic butter

> Sauté onions in 1 Tbsp. of butter until soft and translucent.

> Combine all ingredients (except remaining butter) in a large bowl.

> Form into patties and cook in remaining butter.

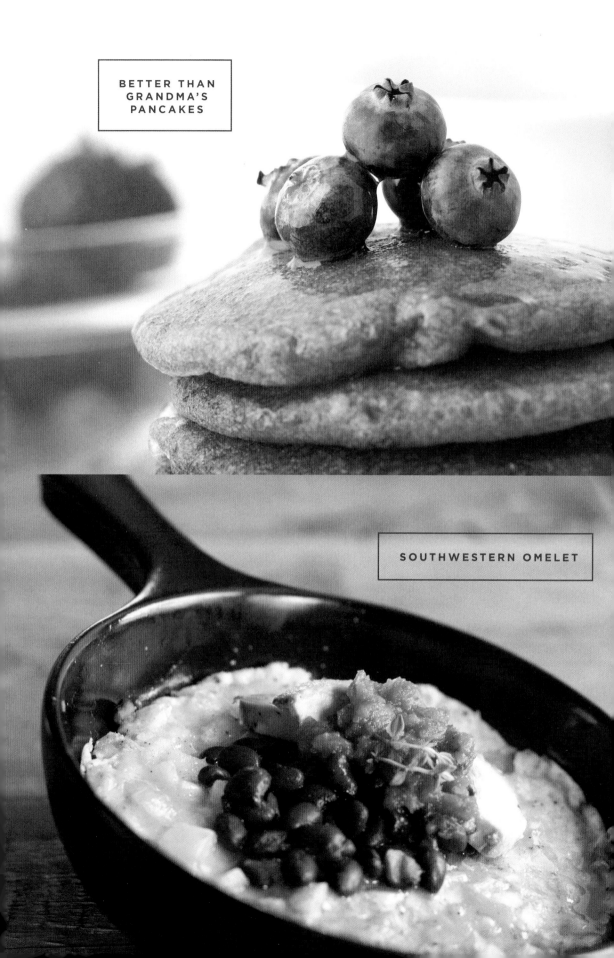

BETTER THAN
GRANDMA'S
PANCAKES

SOUTHWESTERN OMELET

Better Than Grandma's Pancakes

1 c. gluten-free pancake mix

2 eggs

1/4 c. coconut milk

1 scoop protein powder (optional)

1/2 c. berries or applesauce

1/2 tsp. cinnamon

stevia to taste

2 Tbsp. coconut oil or butter

grade B maple syrup

> Mix all ingredients (through stevia) together in a bowl.

> Heat coconut oil or butter in a skillet over medium heat. Drop batter by scant 1/4 cup into pan and cook until done, flipping once.

> Drizzle with grade B maple syrup.

Southwestern Omelet

1 Tbsp. coconut oil

3 eggs

1/4 onion, chopped

1/2 bell pepper, chopped

1 tsp. chili powder

1/4 tsp. black pepper

1/2 c. black beans

1/4 c. guacamole

1/4 c. salsa

> Beat eggs in a small bowl, then stir in onion and bell pepper. Season with chili powder and pepper.

> Heat oil in a large skillet over medium heat and pour in egg mixture. Cook about 3 minutes, or until partially set. Flip with spatula and continue cooking 2-3 minutes.

> Top with salsa, black beans and guacamole before serving.

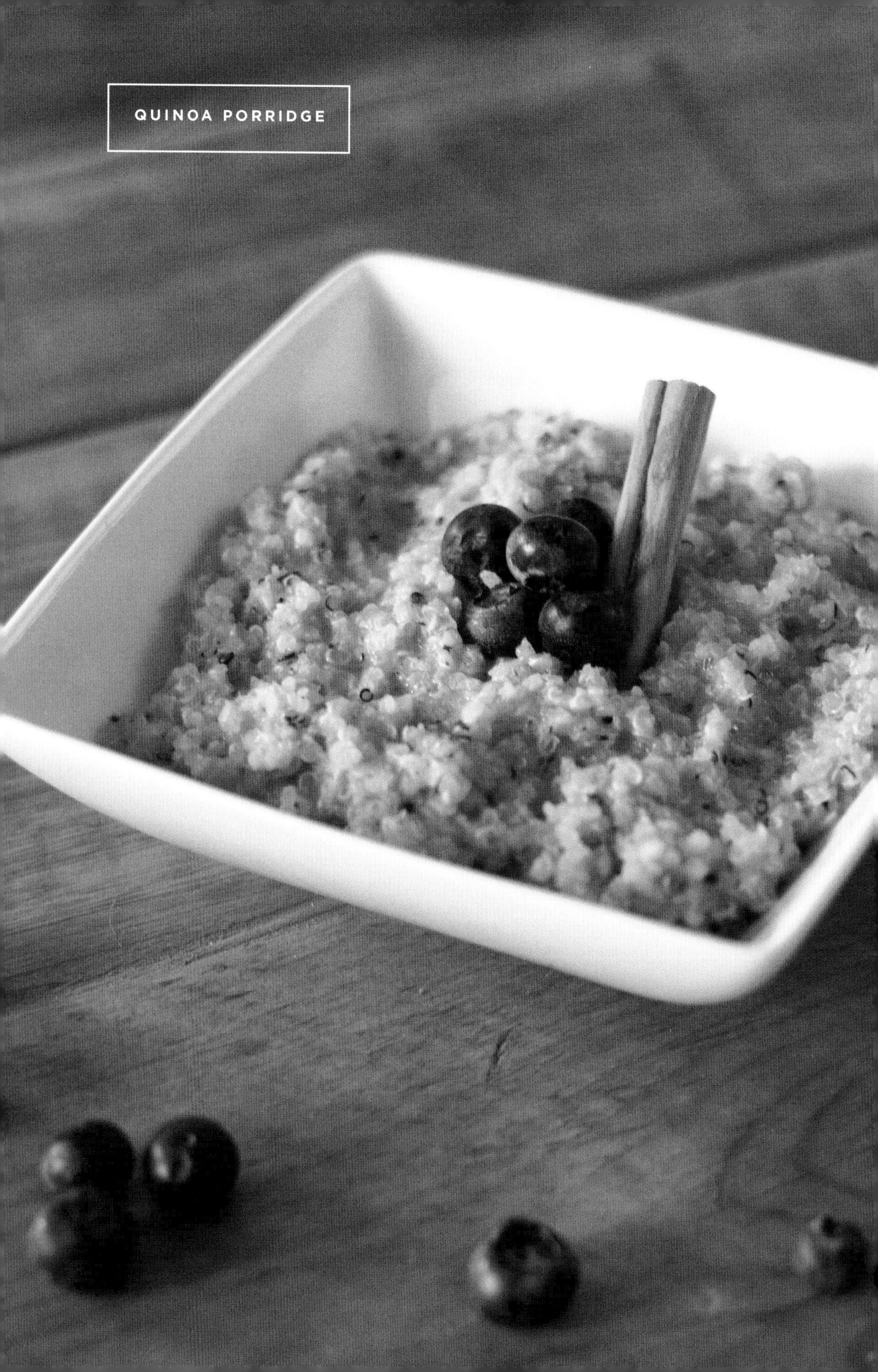
QUINOA PORRIDGE

Quinoa Porridge

1/2 c. quinoa

1/4 tsp. cinnamon

1 1/2 c. almond milk

1/2 c. water

2 Tbsp. honey

1 tsp. vanilla

pinch sea salt

> Heat a saucepan over medium heat. Add quinoa, season with cinnamon and cook until toasted, stirring frequently, about 3 minutes.

> Add almond milk, water, vanilla, honey and sea salt. Bring to a boil, then reduce heat and cook until porridge is thick and grains are tender, about 25 minutes.

> Add more water if needed. Stir occasionally, especially at the end, to prevent burning.

Florentine Omelet

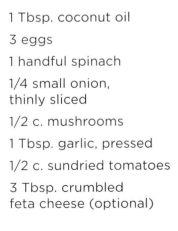

1 Tbsp. coconut oil

3 eggs

1 handful spinach

1/4 small onion, thinly sliced

1/2 c. mushrooms

1 Tbsp. garlic, pressed

1/2 c. sundried tomatoes

3 Tbsp. crumbled feta cheese (optional)

> In a bowl, beat the eggs. Stir in spinach, onion, mushrooms and garlic. Season with sea salt and pepper.

> In a small skillet, heat oil over medium heat. Cook egg mixture about 3 minutes, or until partially set.

> Flip with spatula and continue cooking 2-3 minutes or until done.

> Top with tomatoes and feta cheese.

beverages

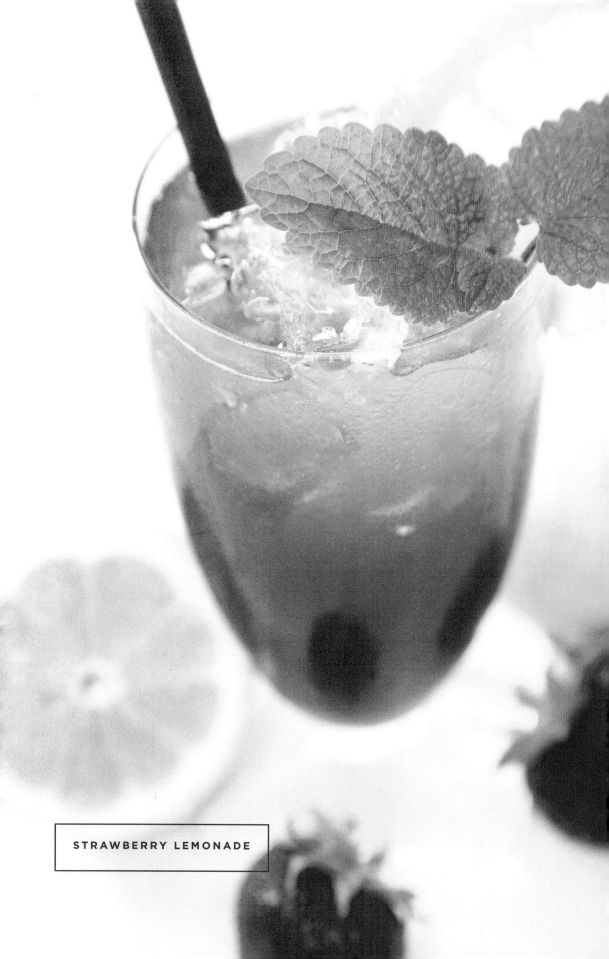

STRAWBERRY LEMONADE

Strawberry Lemonade

3 c. spring or filtered water

1/2-3/4 c. organic
lemon juice

6 organic strawberries,
fresh or frozen

3-4 packets of stevia,
or to taste

> Combine all ingredients in a blender
until smooth.

Refreshing Celery Smoothie

1 apple, cored and sliced

1-2 stalks celery

4-8 strawberries
(fresh or frozen)

Juice from 1/2 organic
lemon

4 oz. water

4-6 ice cubes (if not
using frozen strawberries)

stevia to taste

> Place all ingredients in a blender
and blend on a high setting.

> Serve immediately.

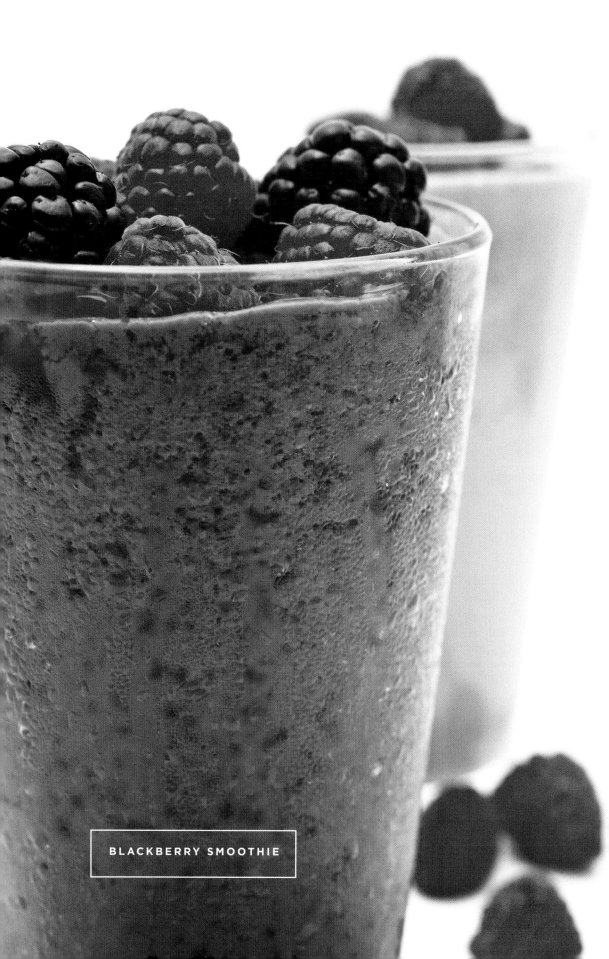

BLACKBERRY SMOOTHIE

Blackberry Smoothie

1 1/2 c. coconut milk
1 1/2 c. frozen blackberries
1/2 c. strawberries
1/2 tsp. lime juice
1/2 tsp. vanilla

> Place all ingredients in a blender and blend until frothy.

> Serve immediately.

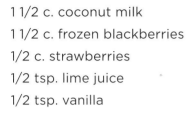

Kale Shake

1/2 bunch kale
1 banana, peeled
1/4 c. red grapes
1 tsp. vanilla
1 tsp. cinnamon
1 dash cayenne pepper
(to taste)
1/2 c. ice
1/2 c. water

> Place all ingredients in a blender and blend until combined.

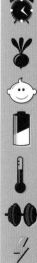

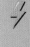

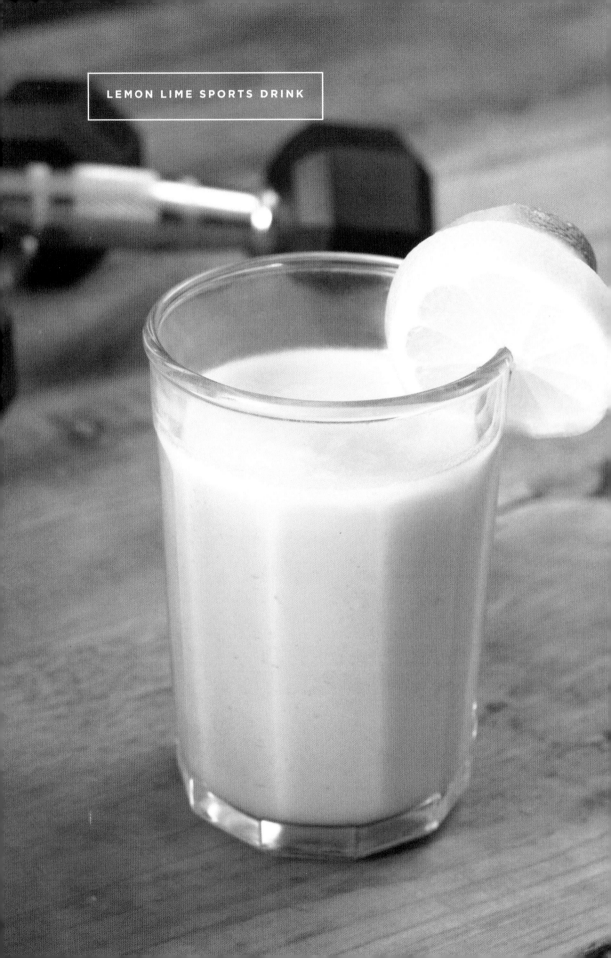

Green Smoothie

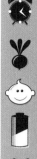

2 bananas, peeled

1 Gala apple, chopped

1 pear, quartered

1 c. kale or spinach

1/2 c. water

> Place all ingredients in a blender and blend until combined.

Lemon Lime Sports Drink

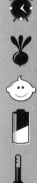

1/2 lemon, peeled
& seeded

1/4 lime, peeled

3 dates

2 c. coconut water

1 Tbsp. honey

1 Tbsp. coconut oil

pinch of sea salt

> Place all ingredients in a blender and blend until desired consistency is reached.

> Serve immediately or keep refrigerated until ready to serve.

GREEN LEMONADE

WATERMELON AGUA FRESCA

Green Lemonade

1 head romaine lettuce

5-6 stalks kale

1-2 apples

1 lemon, peeled

1-2 Tbsp. fresh ginger

> Run each ingredient through a juicer or blend together in a powerful blender.

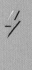

Watermelon Agua Fresca

8 c. watermelon, cut into 2 in. pieces

1 c. water

1 Tbsp. honey

1 Tbsp. fresh lime juice

1 c. Pellegrino

> Blend watermelon, water, honey and lime juice in a blender.

> Stir in Pellegrino just prior to serving.

> Garnish with lime slices and mint leaves if desired.

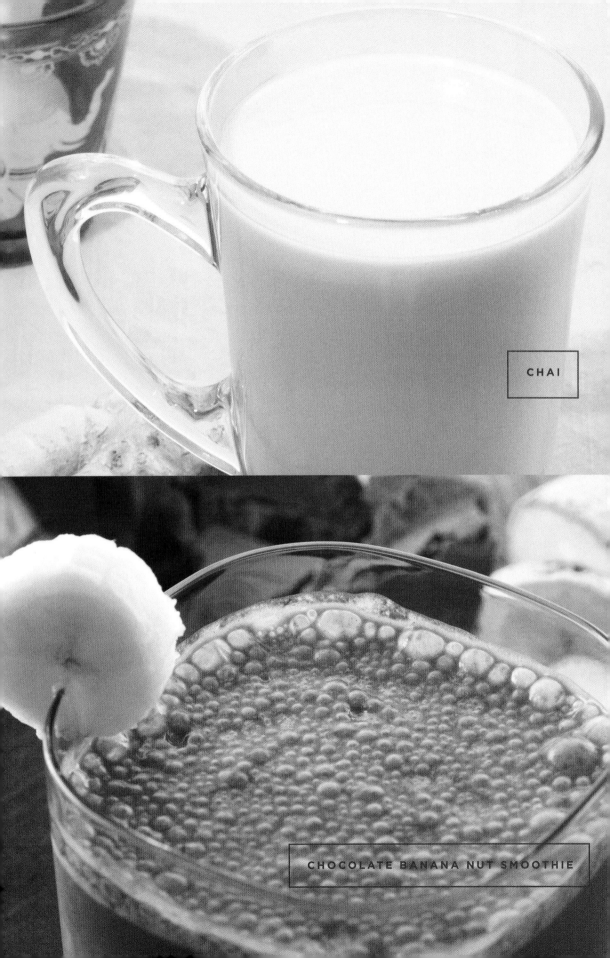

CHAI

CHOCOLATE BANANA NUT SMOOTHIE

Chai

1 c. almond milk

1 Tbsp. grade B maple syrup

sprinkles of nutmeg, cinnamon & clove

> Mix all ingredients in a saucepan and cook over medium heat until warm.

Chocolate Banana Nut Smoothie

1 c. coconut or almond milk

1/3 c. cashew or almond butter

1 banana, peeled

2 Tbsp. unsweetened dark cocoa powder

2 c. ice cubes

stevia to taste

> Place all ingredients in a blender and blend until desired consistency is reached. Serve immediately.

salads

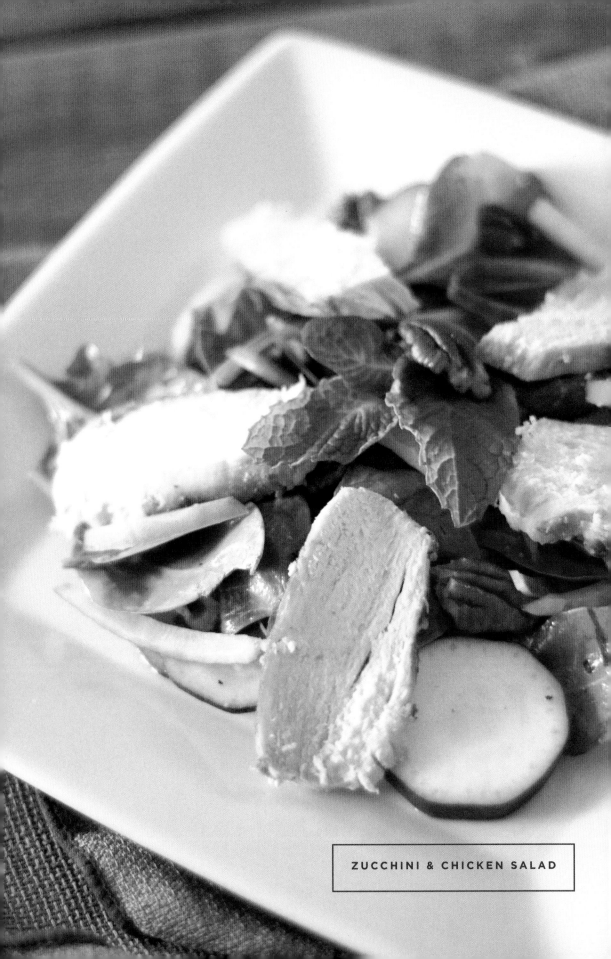

ZUCCHINI & CHICKEN SALAD

Zucchini & Chicken Salad

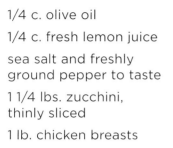

1/4 c. olive oil

1/4 c. fresh lemon juice

sea salt and freshly ground pepper to taste

1 1/4 lbs. zucchini, thinly sliced

1 lb. chicken breasts

1 Tbsp. grapeseed oil

8 oz. spinach leaves, chopped

1/2 red onion, thinly sliced

3/4 c. chopped pecans

1/4 c. chopped fresh mint

> Whisk together olive oil, lemon juice, salt & pepper in a large bowl. Add zucchini and toss to coat. Set aside.

> Heat grapeseed oil in a skillet over medium heat. Season chicken with sea salt & pepper.

> Cook until golden brown on both sides, about 7 minutes per side. Remove from skillet and slice thinly.

> Toss chicken with zucchini mixture, spinach, pecans and mint. Serve immediately.

Not Tuna Salad

1/2 c. raw sunflower seeds, soaked

1/4 c. raw almonds, soaked

2 Tbsp. water

1 Tbsp. fresh lemon juice

1/4 tsp. sea salt

1 1/2 Tbsp. minced celery

1 Tbsp. minced onion

1 Tbsp. parsley

> Place sunflower seeds, almonds, water, lemon juice and sea salt in a food processor or powerful blender and process into a paste.

> Add the remaining ingredients and pulse until just combined.

> Serve as a pate or in between tomato slices and topped with pesto. Will keep in the refrigerator for up to one week.

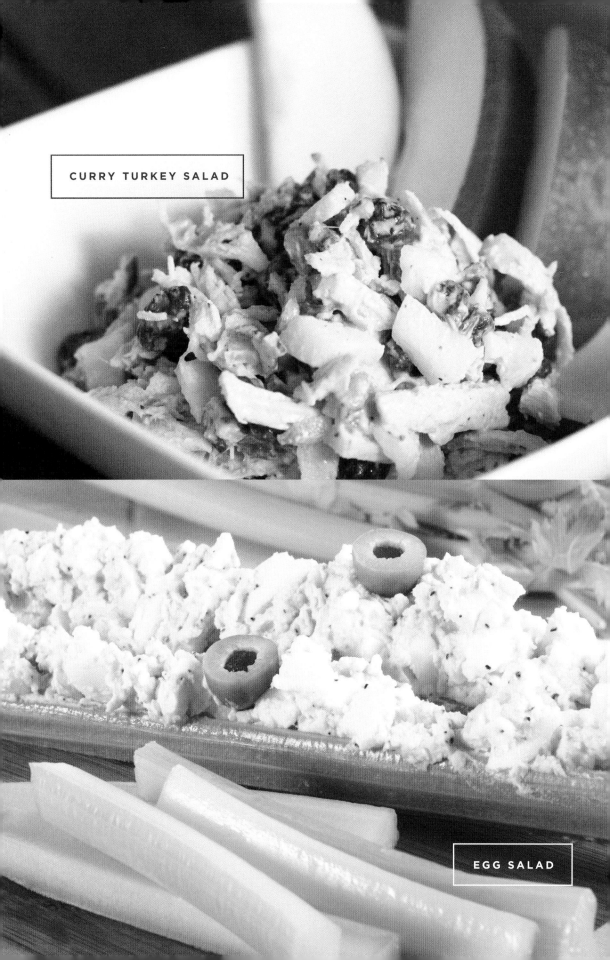

CURRY TURKEY SALAD

EGG SALAD

Curry Turkey Salad

4 turkey or chicken breasts, cooked & diced

1 stalk celery, diced

4 green onions, chopped

1 apple, peeled, cored & diced

2/3 c. golden raisins

1/2 c. chopped pecans

1/8 tsp. ground black pepper

1/2 tsp. curry powder

3/4 c. mayonnaise alternative such as Vegenaise w/ grapeseed oil

> In a large bowl, combine all ingredients. Mix well.

Egg Salad

4 hardboiled eggs, peeled and chopped

1/4 c. mayonnaise alternative, like Vegenaise with grapeseed oil

1 celery stalk, finely chopped

2 tsp. red or sweet white onion, finely chopped

1 1/2 tsp. fresh squeezed lemon juice

freshly ground black pepper & sea salt to taste

> Gently toss eggs and celery together in a medium size bowl.

> In a smaller bowl, combine Vegenaise, lemon juice, onion, salt & pepper. Fold into the egg and celery mixture. Season to taste with salt & pepper.

> Chill for about an hour before serving. Serve over a bed of greens.

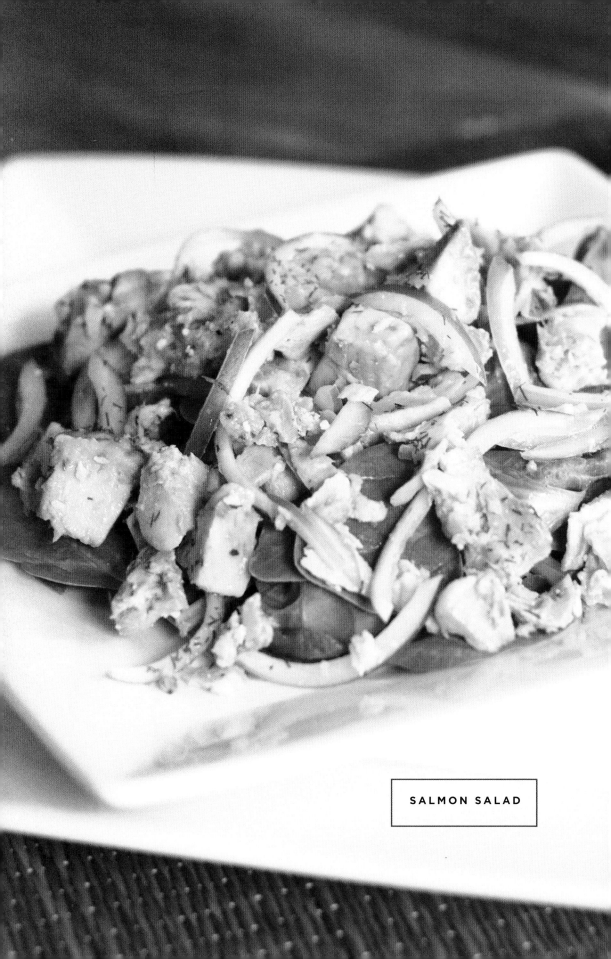

SALMON SALAD

Carrot Raisin Salad

3 c. carrots, peeled
& grated

1/2 c. raisins

1/2 c. homemade
mayonnaise or Vegenaise
w/ grapeseed oil

2 tsp. lemon juice

1/2 tsp. sea salt

1/4 tsp. stevia

1 c. frozen peaches, diced

> Combine all ingredients except frozen peaches in a large bowl.

> Refrigerate until ready to serve. Add frozen peaches just before serving.

Salmon Salad

1 lb. wild caught salmon
fillets or steaks, cooked

1 ripe avocado,
peeled & cubed

1/2 red onion,
thinly sliced

1 Tbsp. fresh lemon juice

2 Tbsp. olive oil

2 Tbsp. chopped herbs
like dill, basil, parsley,
tarragon or chives

sea salt & ground
black pepper

> Break cooked salmon into chunks in a large bowl. Add remaining ingredients and gently toss until combined.

> Refrigerate for half an hour to allow flavors to blend.

> Serve over mixed greens and garnish with lemon wedges.

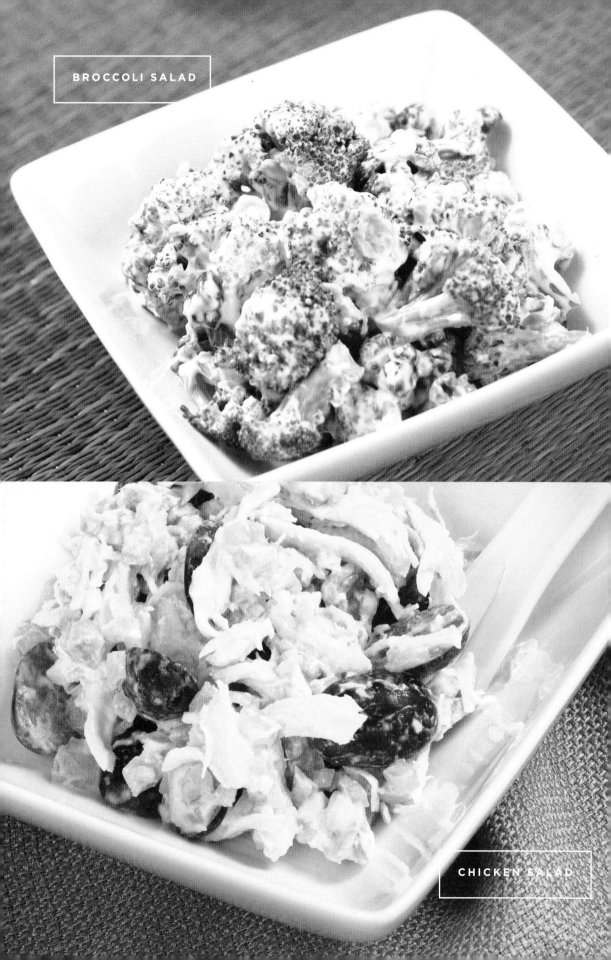

BROCCOLI SALAD

CHICKEN SALAD

Broccoli Salad

1 bunch broccoli

1/2 c. sunflower seeds

1/2 c. raisins

1/2 c. chopped
green onions

3/4 c. mayonnaise
alternative such as
Vegenaise w/ grapeseed oil

2 Tbsp. red wine vinegar

stevia to taste

> Mix all ingredients in a large bowl.

> Refrigerate before serving.

Chicken Salad

3-4 c. leftover,
cooked chicken

2-3 c. coarsely
diced celery

1 c. sliced red grapes

2 tsp. lemon juice

2/3 c. mayonnaise
alternative, such as
Vegenaise w/
grapeseed oil

1/4 c. coarsely
chopped walnuts

sea salt & pepper
to taste

> Place all ingredients in a bowl and
mix together until combined.

CARROT APPLE SALAD

BERRY GOAT
CHEESE SALAD

Carrot Apple Salad

3 carrots, grated

1 apple, cored and grated

1 1/2 Tbsp. olive oil

1-2 Tbsp. lemon juice

sea salt & ground black pepper to taste

> Place carrots and apples in a large bowl. Mix together and set aside.

> In a smaller bowl, whisk together olive oil and lemon juice. Season with sea salt and pepper to taste.

> Drizzle dressing over carrots and apples and toss to combine.

> Serve at room temperature or chill in the refrigerator prior to serving.

Berry Goat Cheese Salad

1 med. red onion, thinly sliced

1 Tbsp. grapeseed oil

12 oz. spring lettuce mix

1/4 c. walnuts, roughly chopped

1/2 c. yellow grape tomatoes, halved

1 c. mixed seasonal berries (strawberries, blackberries, raspberries, blueberries)

4 oz. goat cheese, crumbled

1/2 c. raspberry vinaigrette (see pg 119)

> In a medium bowl, toss onion with grapeseed oil and a pinch of sea salt and black pepper.

> Place on a baking sheet and roast approximately 15-20 minutes at 350 degrees. Set aside to cool.

> In a large bowl, toss spring mix, walnuts, tomatoes, berries, goat cheese, roasted onions and vinaigrette. Serve immediately.

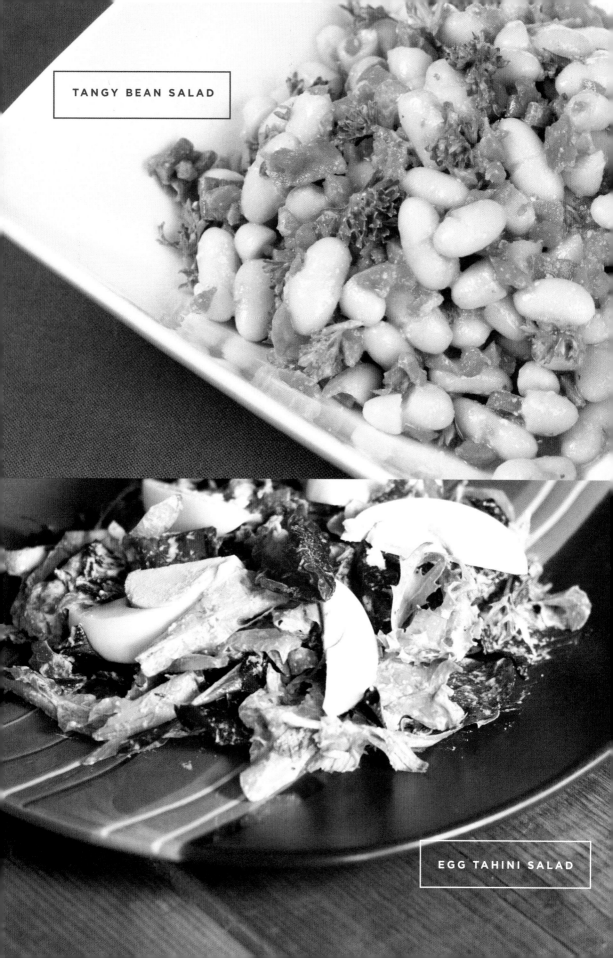

TANGY BEAN SALAD

EGG TAHINI SALAD

Tangy Bean Salad

3 Tbsp. apple cider vinegar

1 Tbsp. Bragg's liquid aminos

1 tsp. stoneground mustard

1 Tbsp. sesame tahini

3 Tbsp. water

2 1/2 c. cooked, drained garbanzo or cannelini beans

1/2 c. thinly sliced green onions

1/2 c. grated carrots

1/2 bunch parsley, chopped

> In a medium bowl, whisk together vinegar, Bragg's, mustard, tahini and water.

> Add beans, green onions, carrots, and parsley and toss to combine.

> Let marinate for 15 minutes before serving.

Egg Tahini Salad

2 heads mixed green lettuce or spinach

1/2 c. sun dried tomatoes

1 med. green onion, sliced

3 Tbsp. tahini

2 Tbsp. apple cider vinegar

1 Tbsp. stoneground mustard

sea salt & pepper to taste

8 hard boiled eggs

> Tear lettuce and place in large serving bowl. Add green onions and sun dried tomatoes.

> In a small bowl, mix tahini, vinegar, mustard, sea salt and pepper. Pour over greens and toss to combine.

> Top salad with chopped hard boiled eggs.

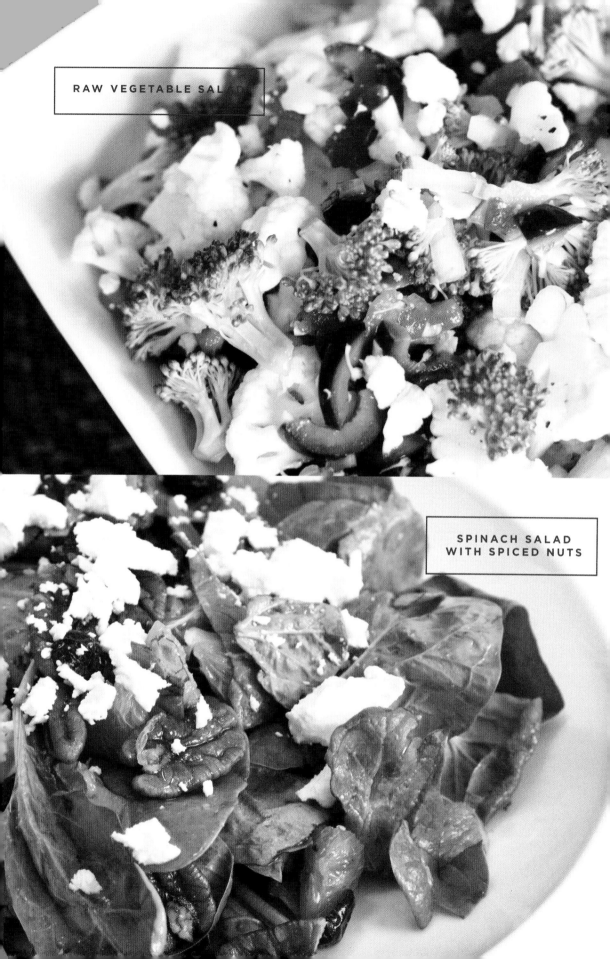

RAW VEGETABLE SALAD

SPINACH SALAD
WITH SPICED NUTS

Raw Vegetable Salad

3 c. cauliflower, sliced

3 c. broccoli, chopped

1/2 c. onion, sliced

1 can black olives, drained

small jar chopped pimento

Dressing:

1/2 c. olive oil

1 tsp. sea salt

3 Tbsp. red wine vinegar

3 Tbsp. lemon juice

1/4 tsp. black pepper

1/2 tsp. garlic powder

> Mix all ingredients together in a large bowl and marinate for at least 4 hours, stirring occasionally.

Spinach Salad with Spiced Nuts

6-9 oz. baby spinach leaves

1 pear, sliced

1/2 c. spiced nuts
(see pg 187)

1/4 c. dried cranberries
or raisins

1/2 c. crumbled goat cheese

> Combine all ingredients in a large bowl.

> Top with Oil & Vinegar dressing (see pg 121).

soups
and
stews

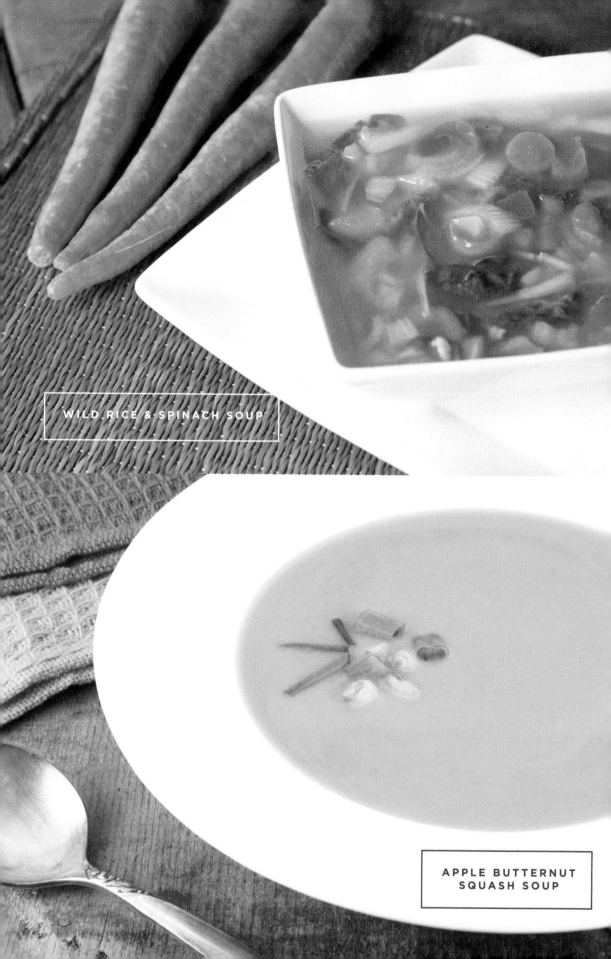

WILD RICE & SPINACH SOUP

APPLE BUTTERNUT
SQUASH SOUP

Wild Rice & Spinach Soup

1/2 c. chopped carrots

1 onion

1 bell pepper

7 oz. baby spinach

1 Tbsp. raw or
organic butter

1 c. wild or brown rice,
cooked

1 quart organic,
free-range chicken broth

1/4 tsp. sea salt

freshly ground pepper

> Chop carrots, onion & peppers and set aside. Coarsely chop spinach.

> Heat butter in a large sauce pot over medium heat. Add rice, onions and bell pepper. Cook 2-3 minutes or until veggies are softened and rice is heated. Stir in chicken broth and cook 5-7 minutes until mixture begins to boil.

> Reduce heat to low, cover and simmer for 15 minutes, stirring occasionally. Stir in carrots, cover and cook an additional 5-10 minutes or until carrots are tender.

> Add spinach, salt & pepper. Cook 1-2 minutes or until spinach is tender.

OPTIONAL: *Add sauteed chicken to the soup before serving.*

Apple Butternut Squash Soup

1 large butternut squash

1 large yellow onion,
chopped

2 Tbsp. grapeseed oil

4 large apples, peeled,
cored & quartered

4 c. vegetable or
chicken stock

1 c. rice milk

1/4 c. coconut milk

1/2 tsp. nutmeg

sea salt

> Peel squash, cut in half and remove seeds. Cut into 2-inch pieces.

> In a large pot over medium heat, sauté onion in grapeseed oil until soft (about 5 minutes). Add squash, apples, stock, rice milk, coconut milk and nutmeg. Cover, bring to a boil, then reduce heat and simmer for 20 minutes, or until squash is tender.

> Pour soup into blender and puree until smooth. Season with sea salt and serve immediately.

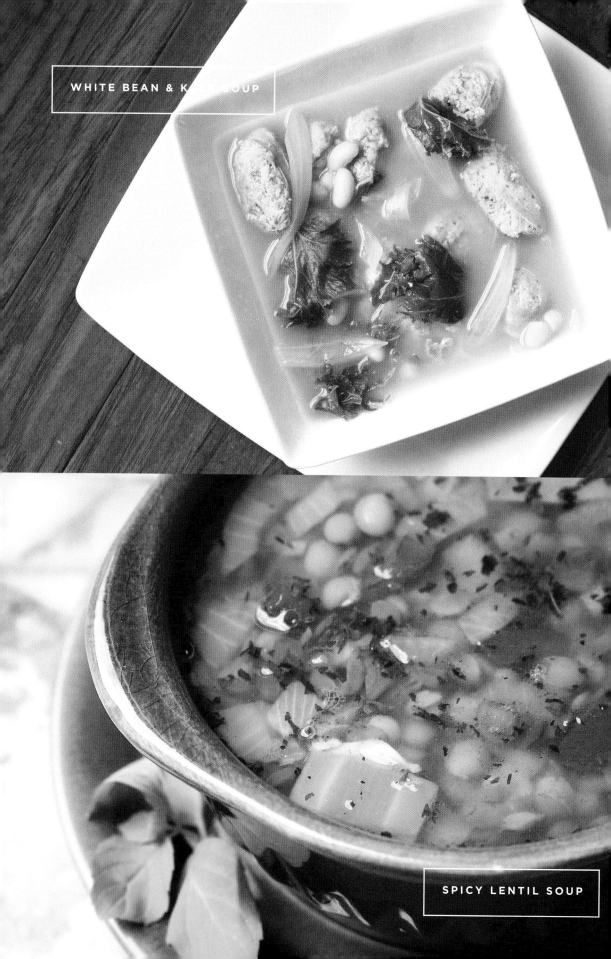

WHITE BEAN & KALE SOUP

SPICY LENTIL SOUP

White Bean & Kale Soup

1 qt. organic, free-range chicken broth

4 links chicken sausage (pork free)

1/2 onion, chopped

sea salt & ground black pepper to taste

4 c. cooked white beans (cannellini, navy or great northern)

1/2 bunch organic kale, stems removed & leaves roughly chopped

1 Tbsp. raw or organic butter

> Heat 1/4 c. broth in a large pot over medium heat. Slice chicken sausage and cook, stirring occasionally, for about 10 minutes. Add onions, sea salt and black pepper and cook an additional 10 minutes.

> Meanwhile, place 2 c. of beans and 1 c. broth in a blender and blend until smooth. Set aside.

> Add remaining broth to sausage mixture and bring to a boil. Add kale, reduce heat, cover and simmer, stirring occasionally, for about 5 minutes.

> Uncover, add beans and bean puree, season with salt and pepper and simmer until hot throughout.

Spicy Lentil Soup

1 Tbsp. grapeseed oil

1 1/2 c. chopped red onion

sea salt & ground pepper to taste

1 (28 oz) can diced tomatoes

1 1/2 c. frozen chopped spinach

2 c. dry red lentils

2 c. water

2 tsp. dried basil

1 1/2 tsp. ground cardamom

1 tsp. ground cumin

> Heat oil in a large pot over medium heat. Cook the onion until golden brown. Season with sea salt and pepper.

> Mix in tomatoes, spinach, lentils and water. Add spices and bring to a boil. Reduce heat to low and simmer for 25 minutes, stirring occasionally, until lentils are tender.

OPTIONAL: *Transfer soup to a blender and blend until smooth or until desired consistency is reached.*

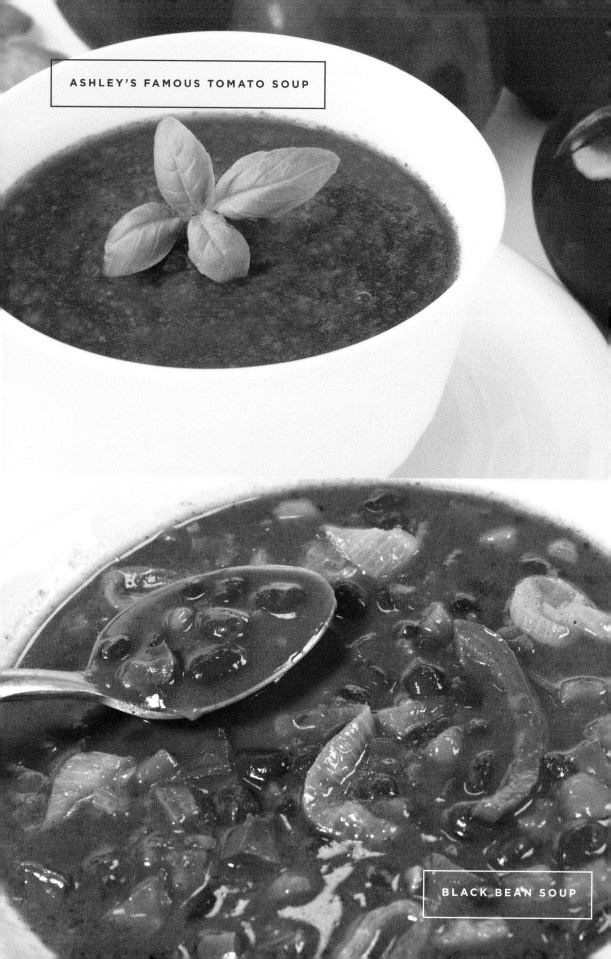

ASHLEY'S FAMOUS TOMATO SOUP

BLACK BEAN SOUP

Ashley's Famous Tomato Soup

2 (6 oz) cans organic tomato paste

15-20 grape tomatoes, diced

3-4 leaves hearts of romaine, finely chopped

1 1/2 Tbsp. cilantro

1 Tbsp. garlic salt

1/4 tsp. cayenne pepper

2 tsp. cumin

1 tsp. black pepper

3-4 c. almond or rice milk

> Warm almond or rice milk in a saucepan over low heat.

> In a separate pot over medium-low heat, simmer tomato paste, tomatoes and chopped romaine for 5 minutes.

> Add cilantro, garlic salt, cayenne pepper, cumin and black pepper. Stir until combined. Simmer for 5 more minutes.

> Add warmed almond or rice milk and let simmer, stirring occasionally, until heated through.

Black Bean Soup

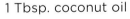

1 Tbsp. coconut oil

2 15 oz. cans organic black beans

1 c. water

1/4 c. chopped white onion

1/4 c. chopped green onions

1/4 c. chopped mushrooms

1/4 c. chopped red pepper

3 cloves garlic, finely chopped

sea salt, chili powder, cumin to taste

> In a food processor or blender, blend 1 can of black beans with 1 cup of water until smooth.

> Heat oil in a large stock pot over medium heat. Sauté onions, mushrooms, pepper and garlic until tender.

> Reduce heat to medium-low, add black bean puree and stir to combine. Add second can of beans, sea salt, chili powder and cumin.

> Heat until desired temperature is reached.

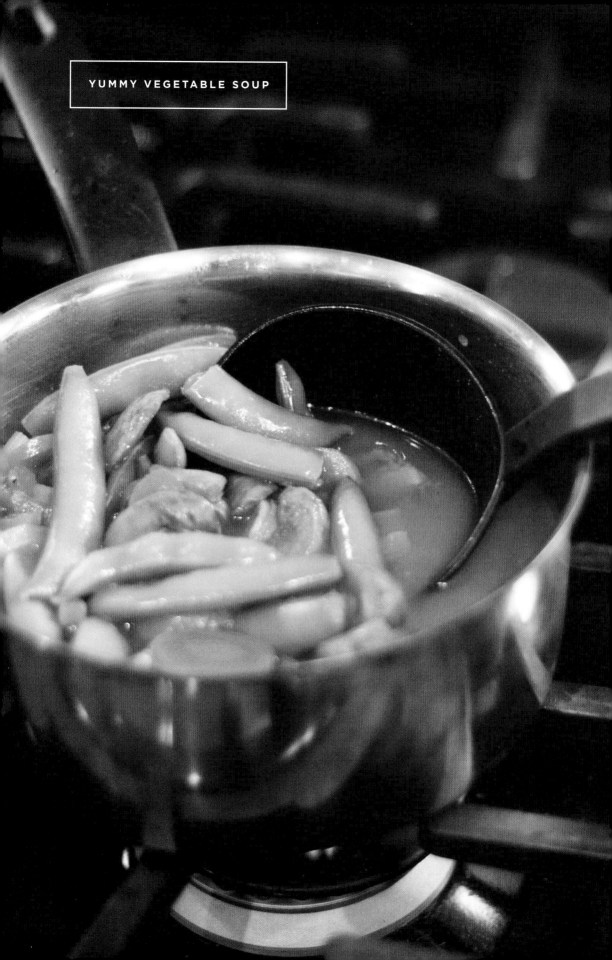

YUMMY VEGETABLE SOUP

Yummy Vegetable Soup

2 Tbsp. raw or organic butter

2 med. garlic cloves, smashed

1/2 c. chopped red onion

1 c. chopped celery

1 large carrot, diced

1 lb. mushrooms, chopped

2 tsp. dried thyme leaves

1 tsp. dried marjoram leaves

1 1/2 tsp. sea salt

1/2 tsp. black pepper

8 c. vegetable or
chicken stock

1 Tbsp. Bragg's liquid aminos

1 10 oz. pkg. frozen
snow peas

1/2 c. chopped parsley

> In a large stock pot over medium heat, melt butter. Add garlic and onions and sauté, stirring occasionally, for 3-5 minutes.

> Add celery, carrots, mushrooms, herbs, salt & pepper. Cover and cook, stirring occasionally, for 7-8 minutes.

> Add stock, cover and let simmer for an additional 10-20 minutes or longer.

> Stir in Bragg's, snow peas and parsley and simmer for a few more minutes.

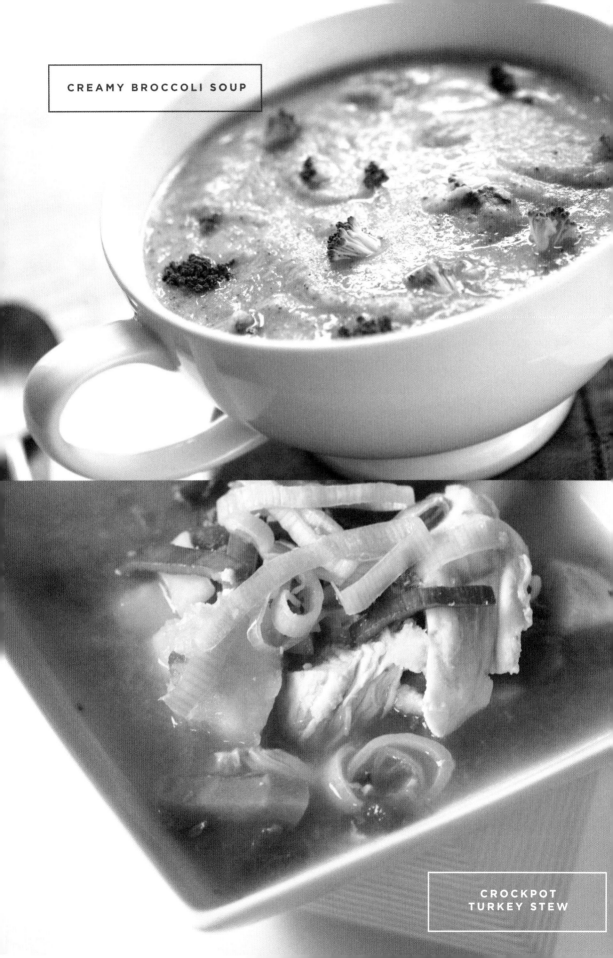

CREAMY BROCCOLI SOUP

CROCKPOT
TURKEY STEW

Creamy Broccoli Soup

2 Tbsp. coconut oil

2 med. green onions, coarsely chopped

2 garlic cloves, minced

2 bunches broccoli

1 Tbsp. basil

2 c. chopped spinach, kale, turnip greens, collards or Swiss chard

2 qt. vegetable or chicken broth

1 14oz. can coconut milk

1 tsp. sea salt

1 Tbsp. curry powder

> Heat oil in a large stock pot over medium heat. Sauté green onions and garlic for 1-2 minutes. Add broccoli and stir until broccoli turns bright green. Add basil and additional chopped greens. Cover and steam for 3-4 minutes, stirring occasionally.

> Transfer vegetables to food processor or blender. Add a little coconut milk and process until smooth.

> Return to stock pot and add remaining ingredients. Reheat gently and stir.

Crockpot Turkey Stew

2 lb. boneless, skinless turkey (breasts, thighs, legs, etc.)

1 med. leek, sliced

2 stalks celery, chopped

2 tsp. thyme leaves

1 tsp. oregano leaves

1 tsp. Italian seasoning

1 c. winter squash, peeled & cubed

1 med. carrot, chopped

1 cinnamon stick

1 16 oz. can organic tomatoes

> Place turkey, leeks, celery and spices into crock pot. Turn on high and sauté until leeks become translucent.

> Add squash, carrots, cinnamon stick, tomatoes, water or stock and simmer, covered, for 2-3 hours on medium or up to 6-8 hours on low.

> Remove cinnamon stick just prior to serving.

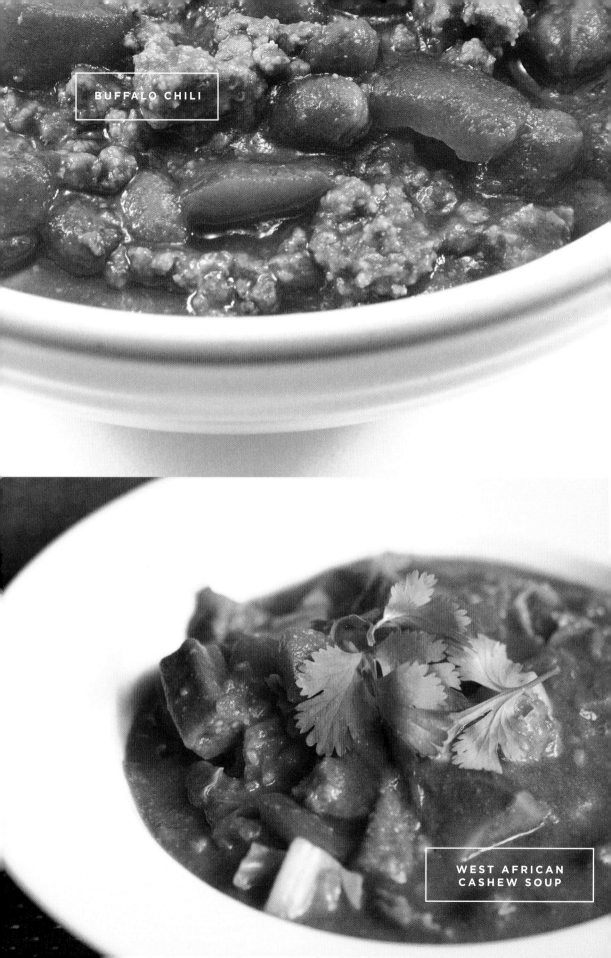

BUFFALO CHILI

WEST AFRICAN
CASHEW SOUP

Buffalo Chili

1 Tbsp. coconut oil

1/2 c. chopped onions

2 garlic cloves, minced

1 1/2 c. chopped celery

1 c. chopped green pepper

1 1/2 lbs. ground bison
or grass-fed beef

2 tsp. thyme leaves

2 tsp. chili powder

2 tsp. cumin

sea salt

1 8oz. can diced tomatoes

1 12oz. jar homemade or
all-natural salsa

> Heat oil in a large skillet or stock pot over medium heat. Sauté onions, garlic, celery and bell pepper until onion is translucent, about 3-4 minutes.

> Add ground meat, thyme, chili powder and cumin and cook, stirring frequently, for 5-6 minutes.

> Add salt, tomatoes and salsa into stock pot or crockpot. Cover, reduce heat and simmer for at least one hour.

West African Cashew Soup

1 Tbsp. toasted sesame oil

1 c. cooked, diced
chicken breast

2/3 c. onion, diced

1 1/2 tsp. garlic, minced

1 1/2 tsp. curry powder

1/2 tsp. sea salt

1/2 tsp. ground black pepper

1/2 tsp. crushed
red pepper flakes

3 c. free range chicken broth

1 (6 oz.) can tomato paste

1 can stewed tomatoes

1/2 c. cashew butter

> Heat sesame oil in a large stock pot over medium heat. Sauté onion until translucent.

> Add seasonings and cook 1 minute more.

> Add chicken, broth, tomato paste, stewed tomatoes and cashew butter. Stir until well combined. Continue cooking until heated through.

sauces
and
dressings

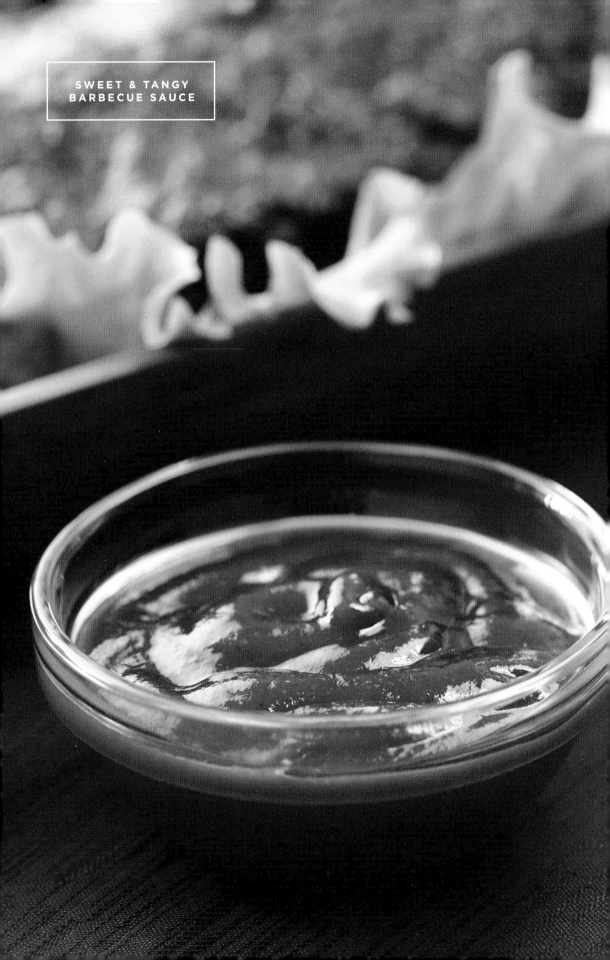

SWEET & TANGY
BARBECUE SAUCE

Sweet & Tangy Barbecue Sauce

2 c. organic tomato sauce

1/2 c. water

1/2 c. balsamic vinegar

1/3 c. honey

1/2 Tbsp. onion powder

1/2 Tbsp. garlic powder

1/2 tsp. sea salt

1 Tbsp. stoneground mustard

1/4 c. Bragg's liquid aminos

> Place all ingredients in a blender and blend until smooth.

> Pour into a medium sauce pan and bring to a boil over medium-high heat.

> Reduce heat and let simmer for 45 minutes.

> Store extra sauce in the refrigerator.

Citrus Dressing

1/3 c. fresh grapefruit juice

2 Tbsp. raw honey

1 tsp. stoneground mustard

3/4 tsp. sea salt

1/4 tsp. freshly ground black pepper

2/3 c. olive oil

> Blend together in a blender.

> Store in refrigerator.

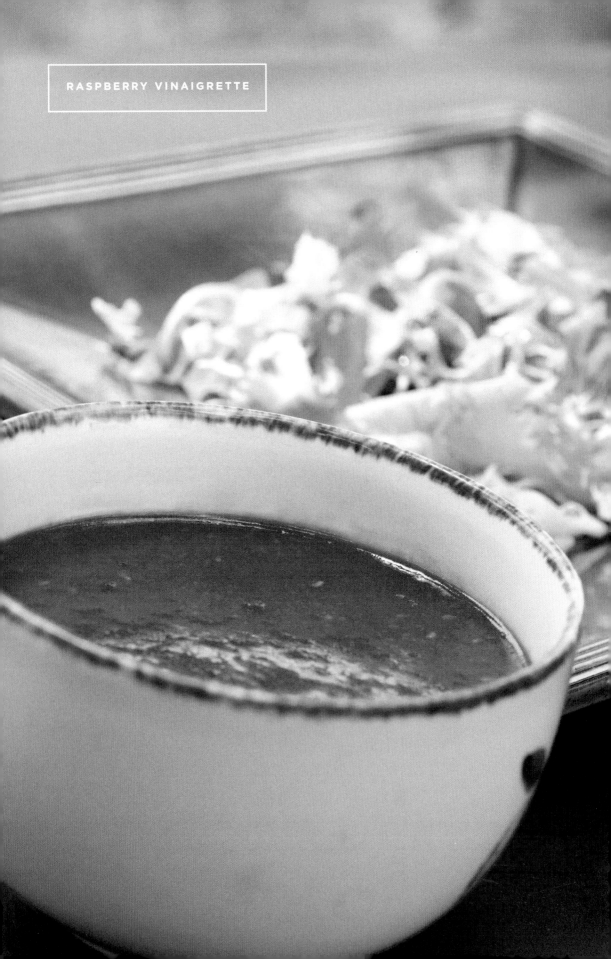

RASPBERRY VINAIGRETTE

Raspberry Vinaigrette

3/4 c. olive oil

1/4 c. apple cider vinegar
or raspberry vinegar

1 tsp. sea salt

2 Tbsp. raw honey

1 tsp. dried basil

1/2 c. fresh or frozen
red raspberries

1/4 c. water

> Place all ingredients in a blender
and blend until desired consistency
is reached.

> Store extra dressing in the
refrigerator for up to 2 weeks.

Italian Dressing

5 Tbsp. red wine vinegar

1/4 c. water

1/2 c. olive oil

pinch of stevia

1/2 tsp. sea salt

1/8 tsp. ground black pepper

1 tsp. stoneground mustard

1 garlic clove, peeled

1/8 tsp. dried basil

1/8 tsp. dried thyme

1/8 tsp. dried oregano

> Place all ingredients in a blender
and blend until desired consistency
is reached.

> Store extra dressing in the
refrigerator for up to 2 weeks.

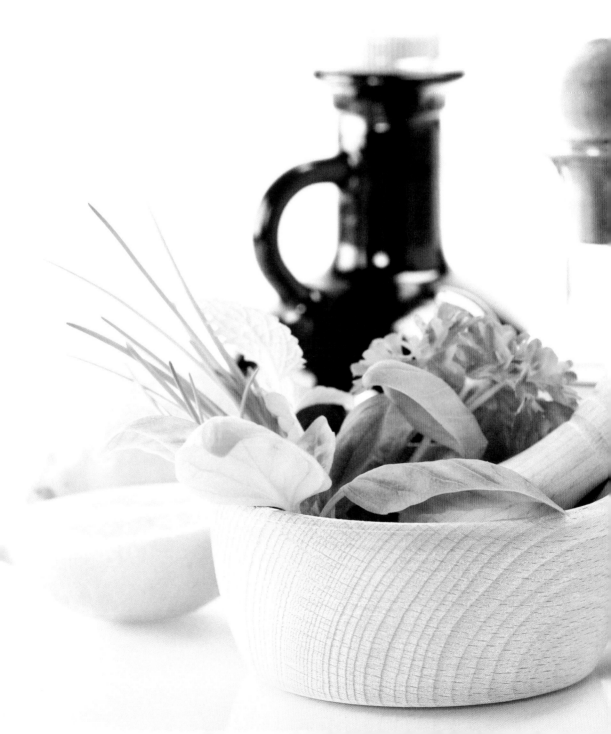

Oil & Vinegar Dressing

1/4 c. balsamic vinegar

1 Tbsp. apple cider vinegar

1 c. extra virgin olive oil

ground black pepper

sea salt

> Combine all ingredients and use as a salad dressing or a marinade for meats or vegetables.

Sun Dried Tomato Pesto

6 cloves garlic

3/4 c. pine nuts

2 c. sun dried tomatoes

1 Tbsp. basil

1 tsp. sea salt

4 Tbsp. olive oil

> Place all ingredients in a powerful blender or food processor and mix until thoroughly combined.

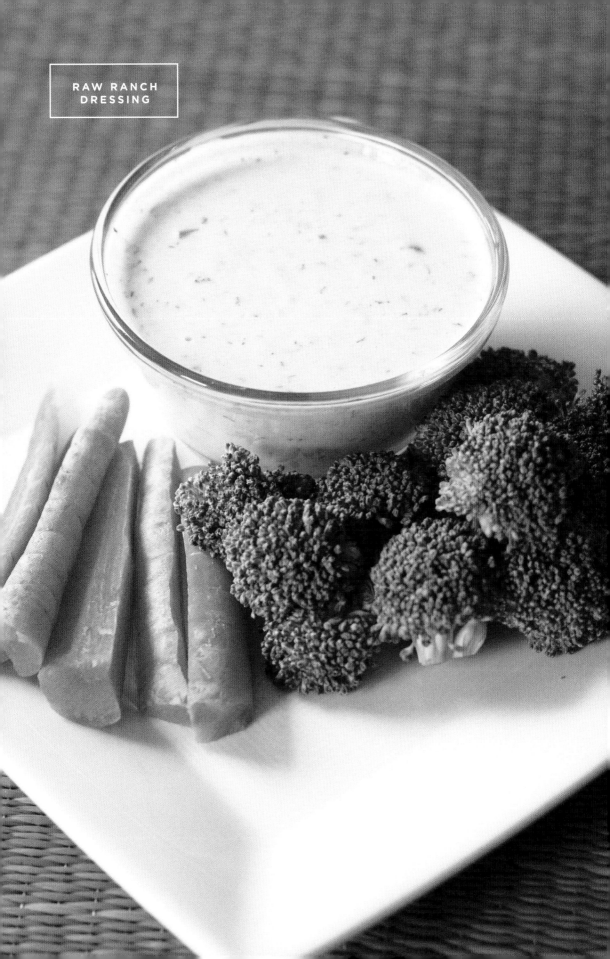

RAW RANCH
DRESSING

Raw Ranch Dressing

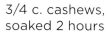

3/4 c. cashews,
soaked 2 hours

1/2 c. water

2 Tbsp. lemon juice

1/4 c. apple cider vinegar

3 Tbsp. olive oil

3 soaked dates

1/2 tsp. sea salt

3 tsp. garlic powder

3 tsp. onion powder

3 Tbsp. fresh basil, minced

3 Tbsp. fresh dill, minced

> Place all ingredients (except the basil & dill) in a blender and blend until creamy.

> Add fresh basil and dill and stir by hand until combined.

Cilantro Pesto

1 c. fresh cilantro leaves

1 large garlic clove

6 Tbsp. melted coconut oil

2 Tbsp. fresh lemon juice

1 c. raw walnuts

> Combine all ingredients in a blender or food processor.

> Serve as a dip or over chicken.

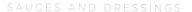

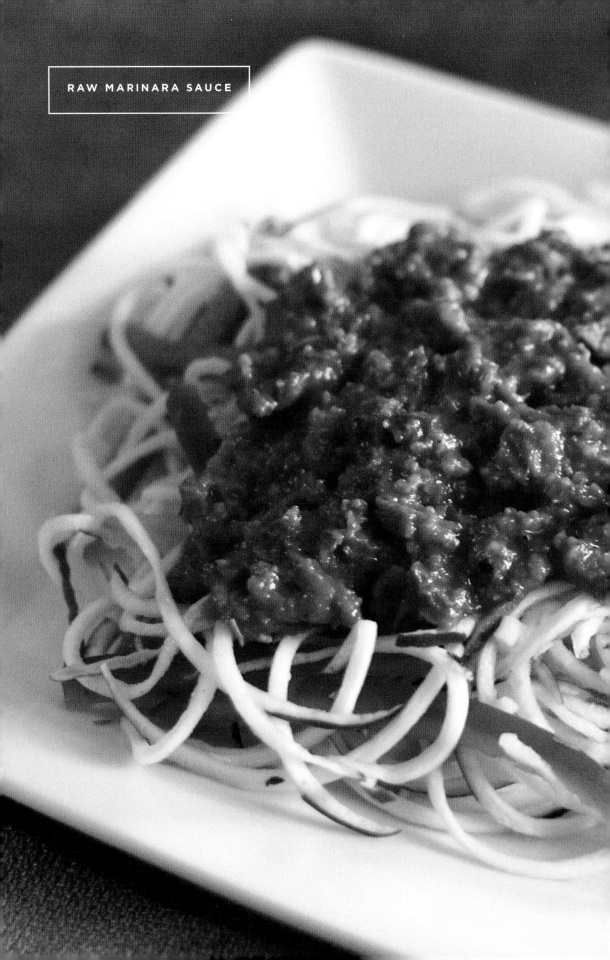

RAW MARINARA SAUCE

Raw Alfredo Sauce

1 c. raw macadamia nuts

1 c. raw cashews

1/2 c. lemon juice

1 1/2 tsp. sea salt

1 Tbsp. minced garlic

1/2 tsp. black pepper

> Place all ingredients in a blender and blend until creamy.

Raw Marinara Sauce

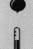

1 ripe tomato

1/2 c. sun-dried tomato, soaked

1/2 red bell pepper, chopped

2 Tbsp. olive oil

1 Tbsp. minced fresh basil

1 tsp. dried oregano

1 garlic clove, crushed

1/4 tsp. + 1/8 tsp. sea salt

dash black pepper

dash cayenne pepper

> Place all ingredients in a food processor or powerful blender and process until smooth.

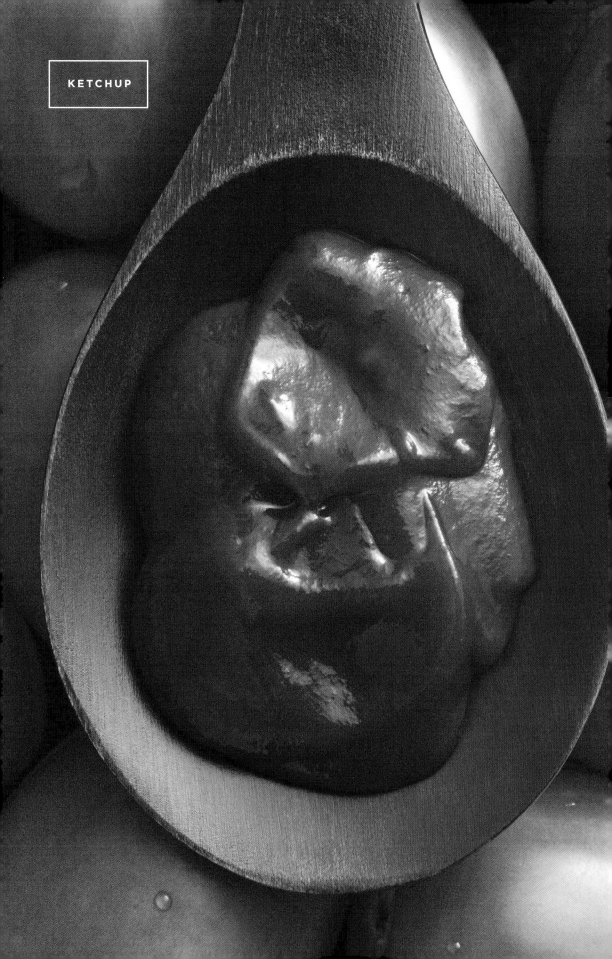
KETCHUP

Ketchup

1/2 c. sun dried tomatoes, soaked 2 hrs.

1/4 c. apple cider vinegar

1/4 c. raisins

1/4 c. onion powder

1 Tbsp. sea salt

> Puree all ingredients in a blender.

> Refrigerate any unused portion.

main
dishes

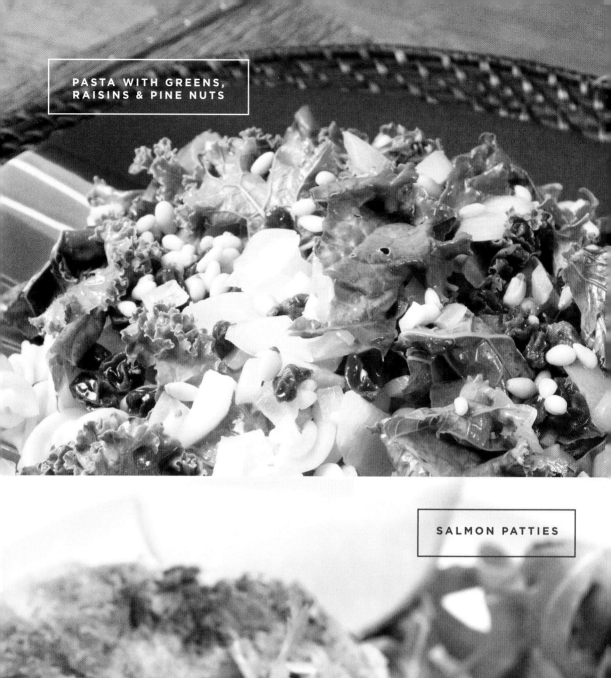

PASTA WITH GREENS, RAISINS & PINE NUTS

SALMON PATTIES

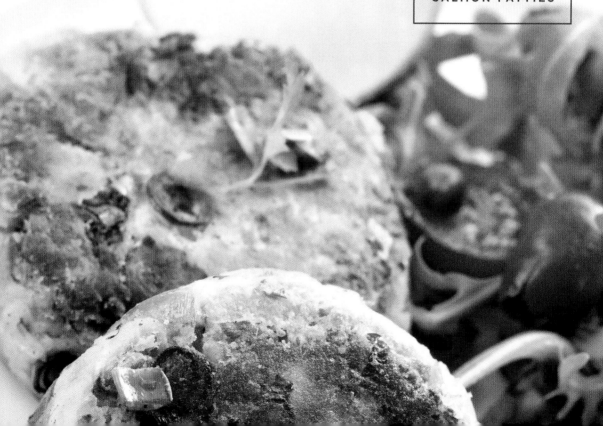

Pasta with Greens, Raisins & Pine Nuts

1/3 c. dark raisins

1/2 c. warm water

4 med. onions, sliced

4 cloves garlic, minced

1 Tbsp. grapeseed oil

1/4 tsp. stevia, or to taste

12 oz. kale leaves, torn

1/2 c. vegetable or chicken broth

1/2 tsp. sea salt

freshly ground pepper to taste

12 oz. sprouted grain or brown rice pasta, cooked & warm

2 Tbsp. pine nuts or slivered almonds

> Soak raisins in warm water for 20 minutes.

> Heat oil in a large skillet over medium heat and sauté the onions and garlic until tender, about 3-5 minutes.

> Stir in stevia and reduce heat to low. Cook, stirring occasionally, for another 10-15 minutes.

> Add kale and broth to the onion mixture. Cover and cook over low heat until the kale is wilted, about 10 minutes.

> Stir in raisins and season with salt and pepper. Spoon mixture over pasta and toss. Garnish with nuts.

Salmon Patties

2 cans wild caught Alaskan salmon

4 eggs

2 Tbsp. olive oil

1/2 onion, chopped

1/2 box Mary's Gone Crackers, crumbled

> Combine all ingredients in a large bowl and form into patties.

> Heat 1 Tbsp. coconut or grapeseed oil in a large skillet over medium heat. Cook patties 5 minutes on each side.

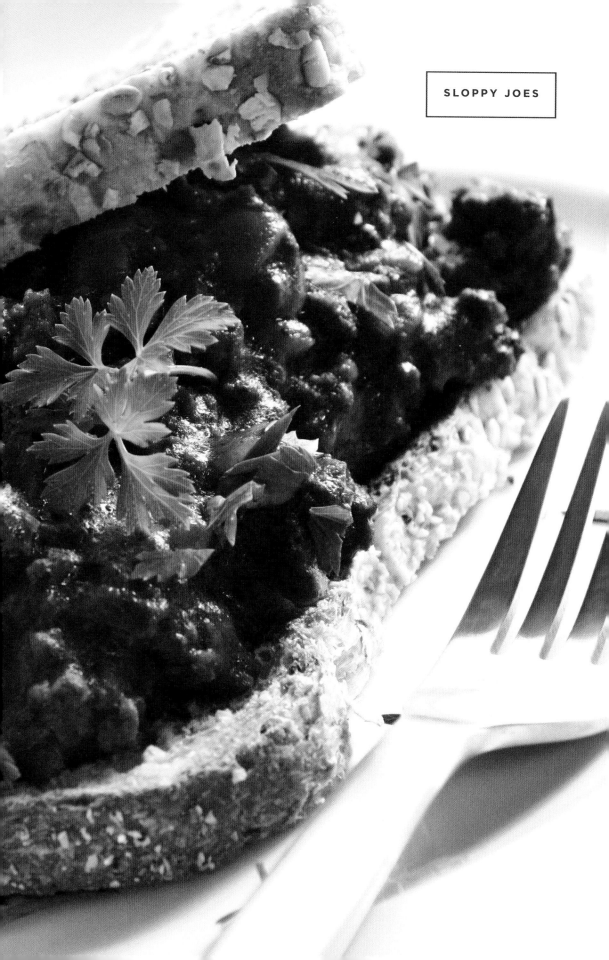

Chicken Sausage with Veggies

4 links chicken sausage (pork free)

1/2 c. fresh broccoli florets

1 green bell pepper, sliced

1 red bell pepper, sliced

1 red onion, sliced

1 Tbsp. grapeseed oil

2 Tbsp. raw or organic butter

garlic powder & black pepper to taste

2 Tbsp. feta cheese (optional)

> Heat oil and butter in a large skillet over medium heat.

> Cut up sausages into slices and cook for about 10 minutes. Add vegetables and cook about 5 minutes more.

> Sprinkle with garlic powder, black pepper and feta cheese.

Sloppy Joes

1 lb. ground turkey or grass-fed beef

1 c. chopped onion

1 Tbsp. grapeseed oil

1/2 c. tomato sauce

1/2 c. sweet & tangy BBQ sauce (see pg 117)

1 tsp. sea salt

> Heat oil in a large skillet over medium heat.

> Sauté onions until translucent, about 2-3 minutes. Add ground meat and cook, stirring frequently, until done.

> Add tomato sauce, BBQ sauce and sea salt. Reduce heat and let simmer for 10 minutes.

> Serve plain or on sprouted grain buns.

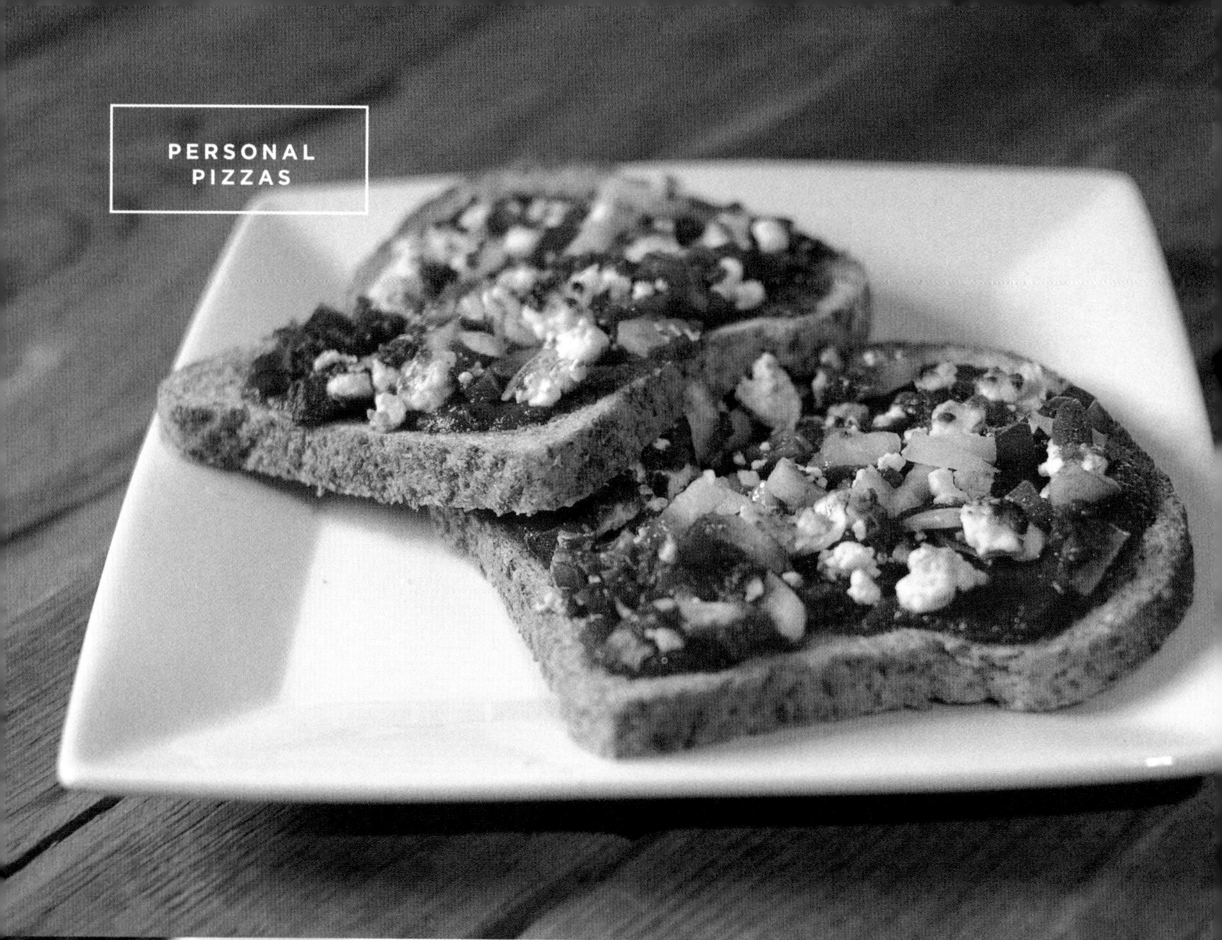

PERSONAL PIZZAS

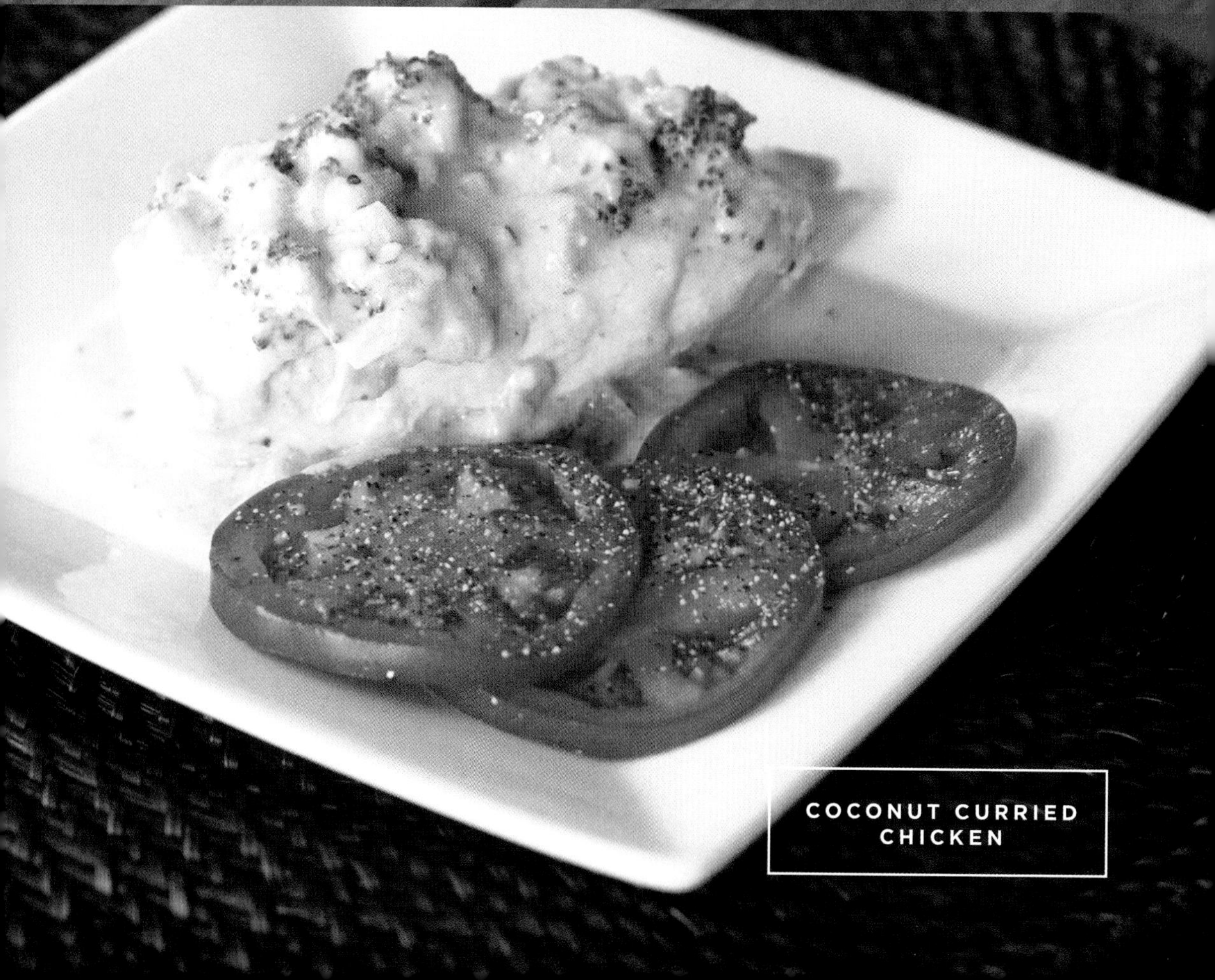

COCONUT CURRIED CHICKEN

Personal Pizzas

2 slices sprouted grain bread

1/4 c. organic pasta sauce

1/4 c. crumbled goat cheese

chopped onion & bell pepper

> Spread sauce on slices of bread.

> Top with cheese and veggies.

> Toast in a toaster oven for 4-5 minutes.

Coconut Curried Chicken

2 lbs. chicken breasts

1 14oz. can coconut milk

2 c. broccoli

1 c. water chesnuts

1 white onion, sliced

2 Tbsp. curry powder

4 cloves garlic, minced

1 tsp. ginger, minced

1 tsp. cinnamon

sea salt to taste

> Heat a large skillet over medium heat and add coconut milk, chicken, broccoli and onion. Cook for 15 minutes.

> Add water chesnuts, curry powder, garlic, ginger, cinnamon and sea salt. Reduce heat to medium-low and cook for 15 minutes more.

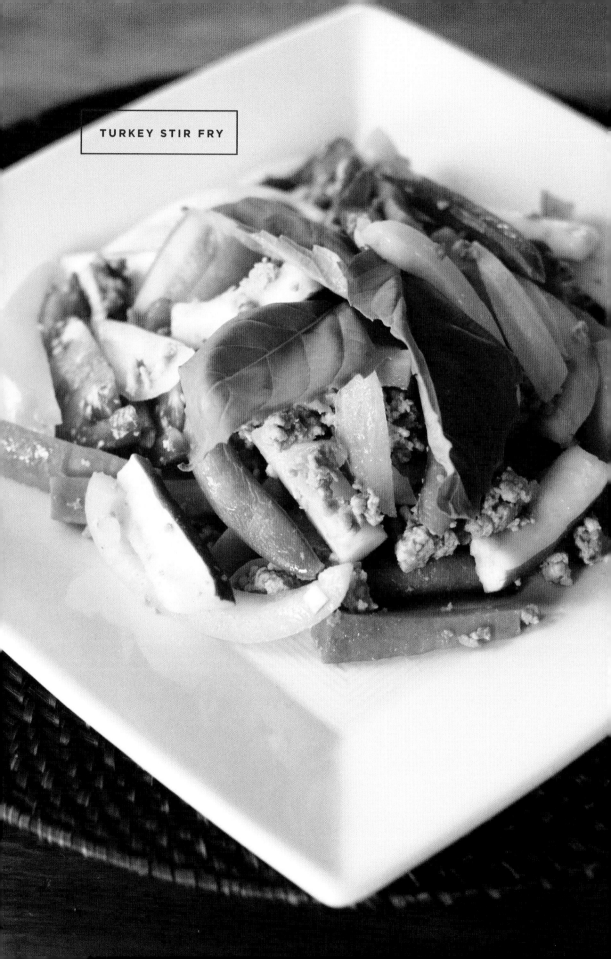

TURKEY STIR FRY

Turkey Stir Fry

2 lbs. ground turkey

3 med. zucchinis, julienne

4 med. carrots, julienne

1 med. onion, cut into
3 wedges

3/4 c. green bell peppers,
julienne

1 garlic clove, minced

1 med. tomato,
cut into wedges

1/2 c. snap peas

1/2 c. broccoli

1 tsp. sea salt

> Heat oil in a large skillet over medium heat. Brown turkey until no longer pink.

> Add vegetables (except tomato) and cook, stirring frequently, for 3-4 minutes, or until crisp-tender.

> Add tomato, salt and cumin. Cook 2 minutes more.

Citrus Marinated Grouper

1-2 lbs. wild caught grouper

1/2 c. fresh lemon juice
(abt. 3 lemons)

1/2 c. fresh lime juice
(abt. 3-4 limes)

1 small red onion,
thinly sliced

2 Tbsp. cilantro, chopped

1 jalapeno pepper,
seeded & diced

sea salt & black pepper
to taste

> Cut fish into bite size pieces and drop into a pot of boiling water for 1 minute.

> Transfer to a shallow dish. Add remaining ingredients and toss to combine.

> Refrigerate for 4-6 hours before serving, stirring occasionally.

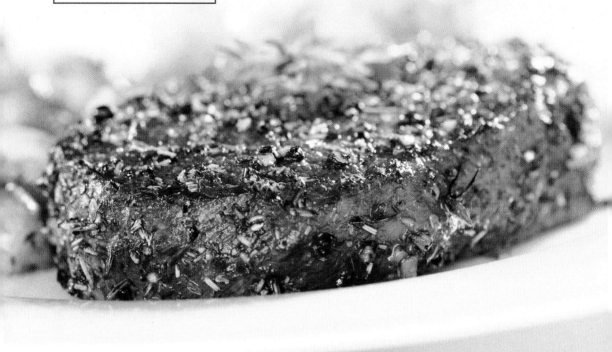

HERB SEASONED STEAK

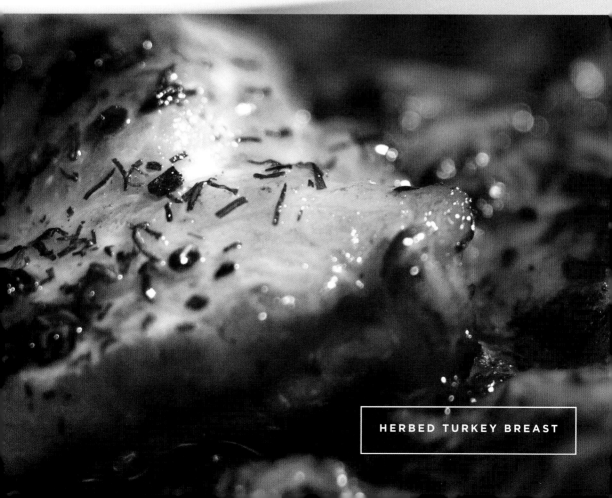

HERBED TURKEY BREAST

Herb Seasoned Steak

2 lbs. grass-fed top steak

4 Tbsp. coconut oil

4 Tbsp. stoneground mustard

4 Tbsp. grated horseradish

4 tsp. dried thyme leaves

2 tsp. ground celery seed

2 tsp. onion powder

2 tsp. sea salt

1 tsp. black pepper

> Rub both sides of steaks with coconut oil.

> Mix mustard and horseradish and spread evenly over both sides of meat. Place on lightly greased broiler pan.

> In a small bowl, mix thyme leaves, celery seed, onion powder, sea salt and pepper. Sprinkle over each side of the meat.

> Broil steaks 3-4 minutes on each side, or until browned on top. Remove to serving platter, let rest 1 minute, then slice and serve.

Herbed Turkey Breast

1/4 c. grapeseed oil

1/8 c. lemon juice

2 Tbsp. Bragg's liquid aminos

2 Tbsp. finely chopped green onions

1 Tbsp. rubbed sage

2 tsp. Italian seasoning

1/4 tsp. black pepper

1 whole turkey breast with bones (5-6 lbs)

> In a small saucepan, combine first 7 ingredients and bring to a boil. Remove from heat.

> Place turkey in a roasting pan and baste with herb mixture.

> Bake, uncovered, at 325 degrees for 1-2 hours, basting every 30 minutes.

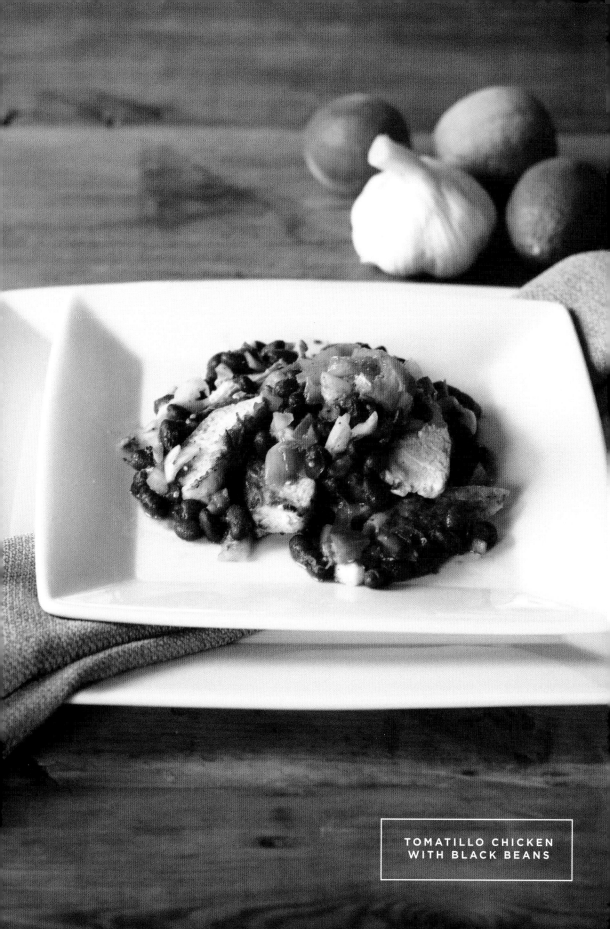

TOMATILLO CHICKEN
WITH BLACK BEANS

Tomatillo Chicken
with Black Beans

1 lb. tomatillos (about 4), cut in half

4 slices (1 inch thick) of a large yellow onion

6 garlic cloves, unpeeled

2 red jalapeno peppers, seeded

4 Tbsp. fresh cilantro

4 tsp. lime juice

1/2 tsp. sea salt

3-4 organic or free-range chicken breasts

2 Tbsp. grapeseed oil

1 tsp. chili powder

> Heat skillet over medium heat and place tomatillos (cut side down), onion slices, garlic and jalapeno in pan. Roast for 5-7 minutes, or until edges are slightly blackened, turning once.

> Remove from heat, cool slightly and peel garlic. Finely chop veggies, garlic and cilantro.

> Combine veggie mixture, lime juice and salt in a small bowl. Mix well and set aside.

> Season chicken with chili pepper and sea salt. Heat oil in same pan over medium heat and cook chicken for 8-10 minutes, turning once. Remove chicken from pan and slice into strips.

> Heat all but 4 Tbsp. of the tomatillo salsa and black beans in the pan. Cook for about 2 minutes or until heated through.

> Spoon bean mixture onto plates. Top with sliced chicken and reserved salsa. Garnish with cilantro leaves.

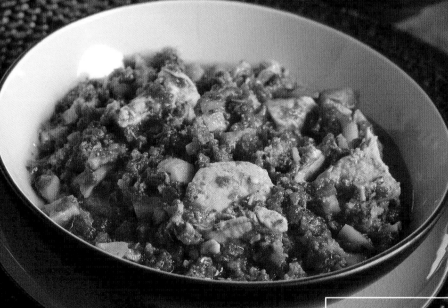

ALMOND ENCRUSTED
SALMON

CROCK POT
CHICKEN & SALSA

Almond Encrusted Salmon

1/2 c. almonds

2 Tbsp. parsley

1 Tbsp. grated lemon zest

1 tsp. sea salt & pepper

4 wild caught salmon fillets

2 Tbsp. grapeseed oil

4 c. spinach

> Grind almonds in a coffee grinder or food processor. Mix almond powder, parsley, lemon zest, sea salt and pepper on a plate.

> Dredge salmon on both sides through the almond mixture.

> Heat oil in a large skillet over medium heat. Add salmon and cook for 5 minutes on each side until cooked throughout.

> Serve over bed of greens and top with fresh lemon juice.

Crock Pot Chicken & Salsa

grapeseed oil

4 chicken breasts
(can be frozen)

1/2 tsp. sea salt

1 jar of all-natural salsa

1 bag frozen organic broccoli

> Wipe crockpot with oil using a napkin to prevent sticking.

> Add chicken, salsa and sea salt. Cook on low heat for 8-10 hours.

> Add broccoli a half hour before serving.

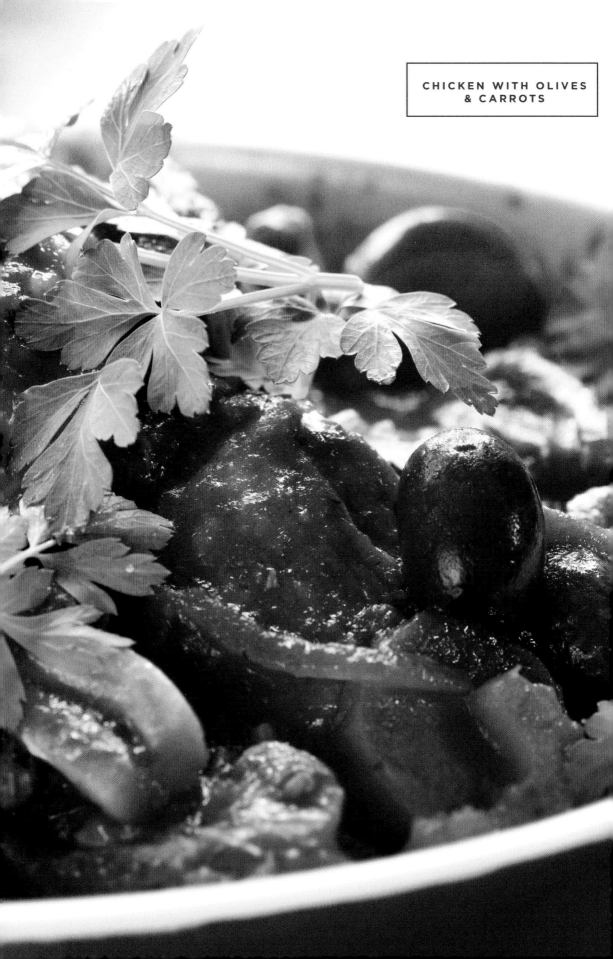

Chicken with Olives & Carrots

2 c. cooked short grain
brown rice, warm

1 Tbsp. grapeseed oil

4 chicken breasts,
cut into small pieces

sea salt & black pepper

1 onion, sliced

2 cloves garlic, minced

1 1/2 c. organic,
free-range chicken broth

4 carrots, cut into
1/2 in. pieces

1/2 c. pitted kalamata olives

1/8 tsp. crushed red pepper

> Heat oil in a large pan over medium heat. Season the chicken with sea salt and black pepper. Cook, stirring occasionally, until chicken is browned, about 8-10 minutes. Transfer to plate and set aside.

> Add onion, garlic and 1/4 tsp. sea salt to the pan and cook, stirring occasionally, for 4-5 minutes.

> Add broth, carrots, olives and crushed red pepper and simmer, covered, until carrots are tender, 8-10 minutes.

> Return chicken to skillet and cook until heated through, 3-4 minutes.

> Serve over brown rice and garnish with parsley.

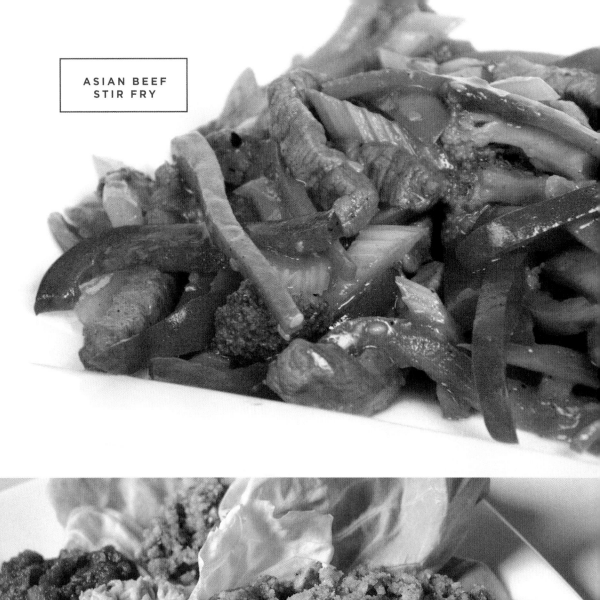

ASIAN BEEF
STIR FRY

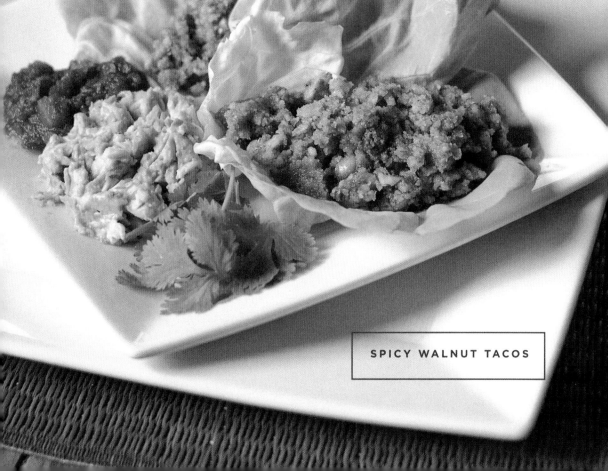

SPICY WALNUT TACOS

Asian Beef Stir Fry

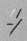

3 Tbsp. Bragg's liquid aminos

2 Tbsp. rice wine vinegar

1 Tbsp. honey

1 Tbsp. grapeseed oil

1 Tbsp. minced fresh ginger root

1 Tbsp. minced garlic

1 lb. grass-fed beef round steak, cut into thin strips

8 oz. snow peas

1 red bell pepper, sliced

> In a small bowl, combine liquid aminos, rice wine vinegar and honey and set aside.

> Heat oil in a large skillet over medium heat. Stir-fry ginger and garlic for about 30 seconds.

> Add steak and stir-fry for 2 minutes or until evenly browned. Add snow peas and red bell pepper and cook for an additional 3 minutes.

> Add sauce and bring to a boil, stirring constantly. Lower heat and simmer for a few more minutes.

> Serve over brown rice.

Spicy Walnut Tacos

1 1/2 c. raw walnuts, ground in food processor

1 1/2 tsp. ground cumin

3/4 tsp. coriander

2 tsp. Bragg's liquid aminos

pinch of cayenne pepper

> Mix all ingredients in a food processor until it is a coarse mixture.

> Serve in lettuce wraps with salsa and guacamole.

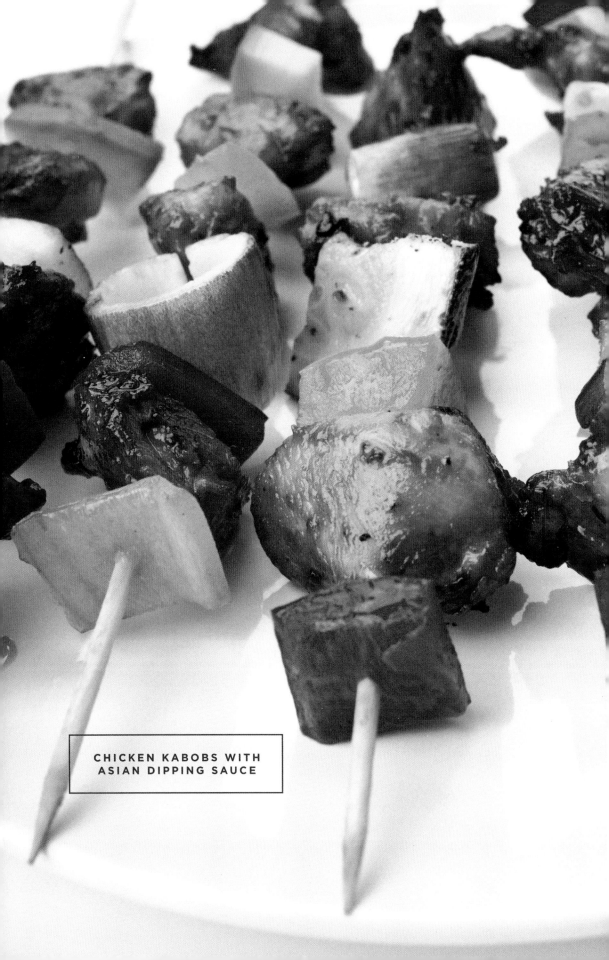

CHICKEN KABOBS WITH
ASIAN DIPPING SAUCE

Chicken Kabobs with
Asian Dipping Sauce

2 lbs. chicken breasts,
cut into cubes

1/2 red onion, chopped
in large pieces

1-2 bell peppers,
chopped in large pieces

8 oz. button mushrooms,
cut in half

> Soak kabob sticks in water for
at least 2 hours.

> Slide meat and vegetables
onto kabobs.

> Grill or broil until done.

Sauce:

1 Tbsp. honey

4 Tbsp. cashew butter

2 Tbsp. fresh lime juice

1 tsp. fresh minced ginger

1 clove garlic, minced

1/2 c. coconut milk

2 Tbsp. Bragg's liquid aminos

1 Tbsp. water

crushed red pepper to taste

> Place all ingredients into a
blender and blend until thoroughly
combined.

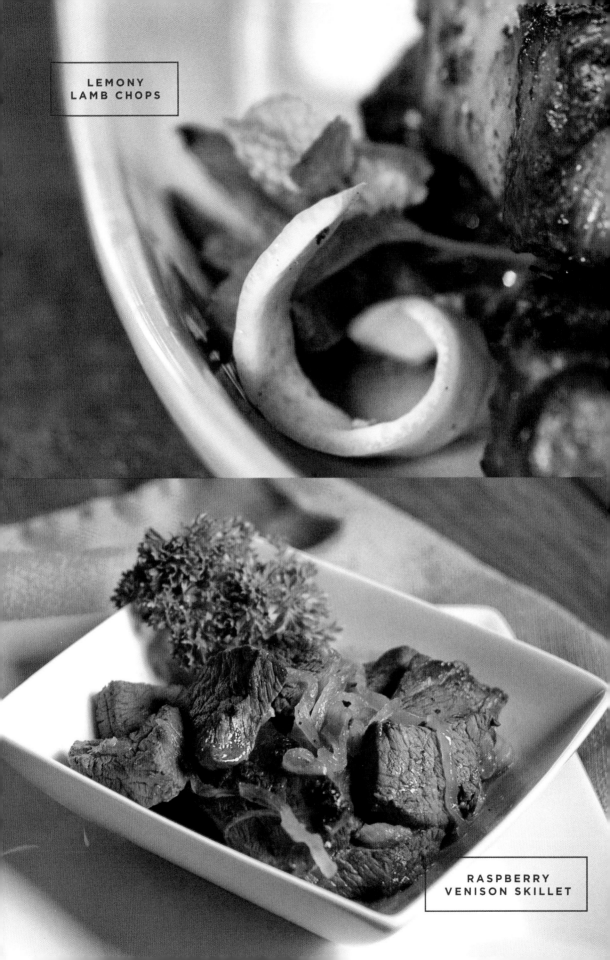

LEMONY
LAMB CHOPS

RASPBERRY
VENISON SKILLET

Lemony Lamb Chops

4 grass-fed lamb chops
(loin, rib or shoulder)

1 tsp. grated lemon zest

1/2 tsp. dried rosemary,
crushed

1 tsp. oregano

1 tsp. tarragon

1 Tbsp. lemon juice

1 Tbsp. Bragg's liquid
aminos

> Combine lemon zest, herbs, lemon juice and aminos in a small bowl to make a paste.

> Spread on lamb and broil 3-4 minutes per side. Be careful not to overcook.

Raspberry Venison Skillet

3/4 c. raspberry vinaigrette
(see pg 119)

2 Tbsp. maple syrup

2 Tbsp. Bragg's liquid aminos

2 lbs. venison, cut into
1/2 inch strips

2 Tbsp. organic butter

2 Tbsp. grapeseed oil

3/4 c. water

2 sweet onions, thinly sliced

1 Tbsp. minced garlic

sea salt & ground pepper
to taste

1/2 tsp. stevia

> Whisk together the vinaigrette, maple syrup and liquid aminos in a large bowl. Stir in the venison until well coated and set aside.

> In a large skillet over medium high heat, add the butter, grapeseed oil, water, onions and garlic. Cook, stirring frequently, until the onions have caramelized, about 10 minutes. Stir in stevia and cook 2-3 minutes more.

> Add the venison and marinade to the skillet and cook until venison is no longer pink in the center, about 5 minutes.

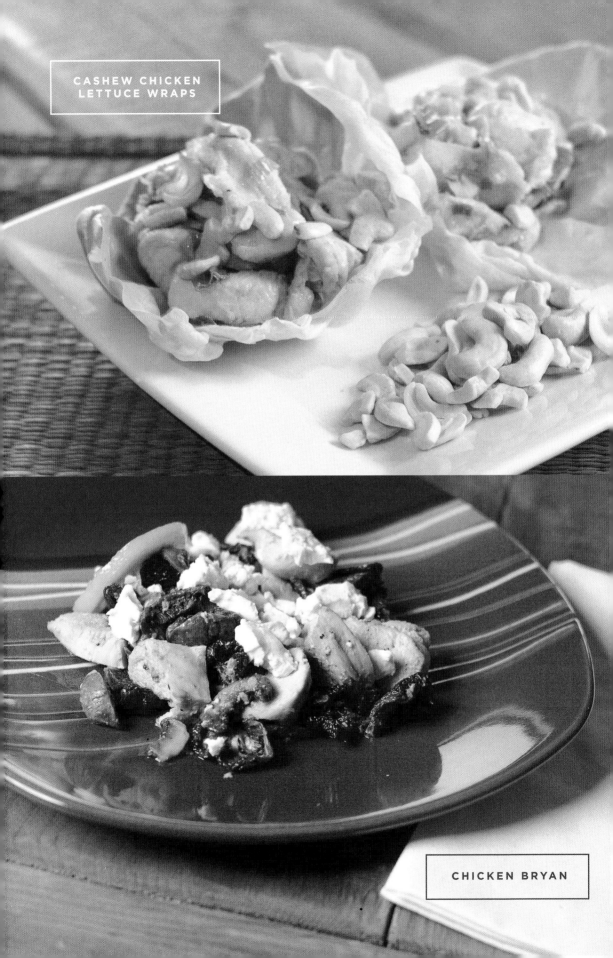

CASHEW CHICKEN
LETTUCE WRAPS

CHICKEN BRYAN

Cashew Chicken Lettuce Wraps

2 Tbsp. Bragg's liquid aminos

2 Tbsp. honey

2 Tbsp. grapeseed oil

1 1/2 lbs. chicken breasts, cut into 3/4 in. pieces

sea salt & pepper to taste

2 cloves garlic, finely chopped

1 Tbsp. grated ginger root

1 bunch scallions, trimmed & sliced

1 8oz. can sliced water chesnuts, drained

1/4 c. cashews, toasted

> Combine aminos and honey in a small bowl and set aside.

> Heat oil in a large skillet over medium heat. Season chicken with sea salt and pepper and cook, stirring occasionally, until chicken begins to brown, about 5 minutes.

> Stir in garlic, ginger and scallions and cook for 1 minute.

> Stir in water chesnuts and sauce. Continue to cook until chicken is cooked through, about 4 minutes. Remove from heat and sprinkle with cashews.

> Divide lettuce leaves among individual plates and spoon chicken over the top.

Chicken Bryan

4 Tbsp. grapeseed oil

2 lbs. chicken breasts

1 lemon, sliced

6 cloves garlic, minced

2 c. mushrooms

2 c. sun dried tomatoes

1/2 c. goat cheese

1 Tbsp. basil

1/2 tsp. sea salt

1/2 c. raw or organic butter

> Heat oil in a large skillet over medium heat. Add chicken and minced garlic and cook for 8 minutes.

> Add butter and lemon slices to the pan. Flip chicken and cook for 5 more minutes.

> Add mushrooms, sun dried tomatoes, basil and sea salt.

> Top chicken with goat cheese, reduce heat and cover pan for 2 minutes.

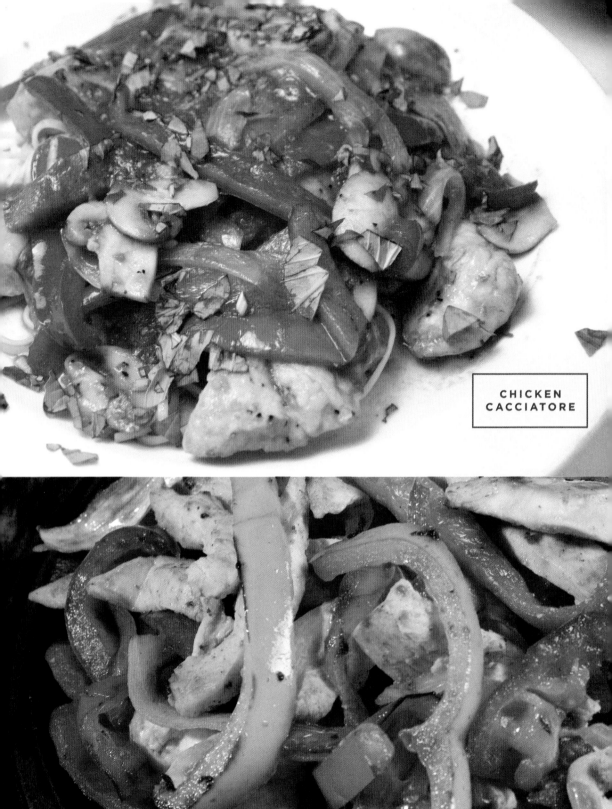

CHICKEN
CACCIATORE

CHICKEN FAJITAS

Chicken Cacciatore

1 Tbsp. grapeseed oil

2 lbs. chicken breasts

2 large tomatoes, chopped

1 large onion, thinly sliced

2 c. sliced mushrooms

3/4 c. red wine

3 garlic cloves, minced

sea salt & Italian
seasoning to taste

> Heat oil in a large skillet over medium heat. Add chicken, onion, garlic and red wine and cook for 15 minutes, turning chicken once.

> Reduce heat to medium-low. Add mushrooms, tomatoes, sea salt and Italian seasoning. Cook until chicken is done and vegetables are tender.

Chicken Fajitas

2 lbs. chicken breast

2 Tbsp. coconut oil

1 green bell pepper

1 red bell pepper

1 white onion

2 cloves garlic,
finely chopped

1 tsp. sea salt

1 tsp. cumin

1 tsp. chili powder

1 can organic black beans

1 package sprouted grain
or brown rice tortillas

> Heat oil in a large skillet over medium heat. Add chicken breast. Sprinkle with 1/2 tsp. sea salt and garlic and cook until done. Remove from heat and let cool. Using a knife and fork, pull apart chicken until shredded.

> In the same skillet, add enough water to cover the bottom of the pan. Add sliced bell peppers and onion. Add remaining garlic and sea salt and cook for 5-10 minutes.

> Add chicken back to skillet and season with cumin and chili powder. Cook until veggies are tender.

> Serve over tortillas with black beans.

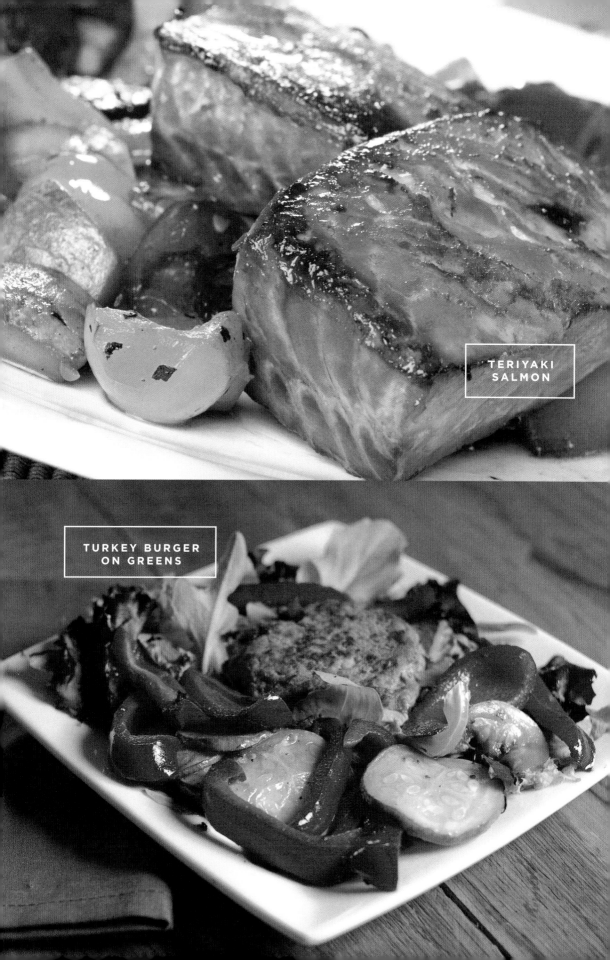

TERIYAKI
SALMON

TURKEY BURGER
ON GREENS

Teriyaki Salmon

1/4 c. grapeseed oil

1/4 c. fresh lemon juice

1/4 c. Bragg's liquid aminos

1 tsp. stoneground mustard

1 tsp. ground ginger

1/4 tsp. garlic powder

4 wild caught salmon steaks

> In a storage bag, combine first 6 ingredients and mix well. Set aside 1/4 c. of marinade in the refrigerator for basting. Add salmon to the bag and place in refrigerator to marinate for 1 hour.

> Drain and discard marinade. Broil or grill salmon for 4-5 minutes each side. Brush with reserved marinade.

Turkey Burger on Greens

2 lbs. ground turkey

2 zucchinis, sliced

3 red bell peppers, cut into strips

4 green onions, chopped

2 tsp. Bragg's liquid aminos

2 tsp. cumin

2 tsp. curry powder

sea salt & black pepper to taste

1 Tbsp. grapeseed oil

> Place ground turkey in a large mixing bowl and mix with Bragg's, 1 tsp. cumin, 1 tsp. curry powder, sea salt and pepper. Form into patties.

> Heat oil in a large skillet over medium heat and cook burgers until done. Remove to baking dish to keep warm in the oven. Sauté vegetables in same pan for 3-4 minutes, adding more oil if necessary.

> Add chicken back to skillet and season with remaining cumin and curry powder. Cook until veggies are tender.

> Serve burgers over a bed of greens and top with veggies.

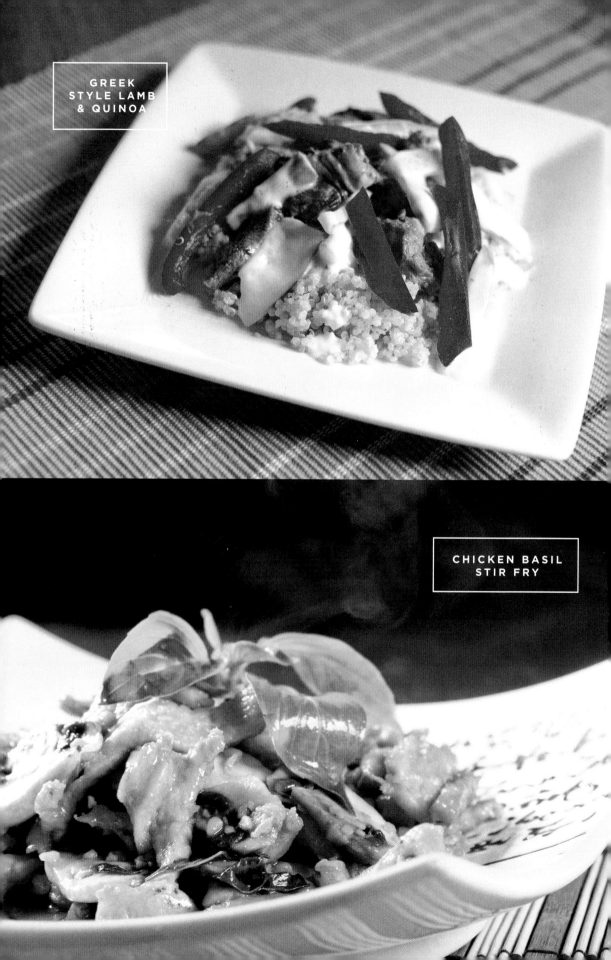

GREEK
STYLE LAMB
& QUINOA

CHICKEN BASIL
STIR FRY

Greek Style Lamb & Quinoa

1 lb. boneless leg of lamb, trimmed & thinly sliced

2 Tbsp. chopped fresh oregano, divided

3 tsp. lemon juice, divided

2 cloves garlic, minced

sea salt & black pepper to taste

1 Tbsp. grapeseed oil, divided

1/2 c. goat's milk yogurt

1/2 cucumber, seeded & grated

4 c. cooked quinoa

1 red bell pepper, chopped

> Place lamb, half the oregano, half the lemon juice, garlic, 1 tsp. sea salt and 1/4 tsp. pepper in a large bowl and toss together.

> Heat oil in a large skillet over medium heat. Add lamb and cook, stirring frequently, until cooked through, about 5-7 minutes.

> In a medium bowl, mix together yogurt, cucumber, remaining lemon juice, sea salt and pepper to taste.

> Serve lamb on top of cooked quinoa, drizzle with sauce and top with chopped bell peppers and remaining oregano.

Chicken Basil Stir Fry

1 Tbsp. grapeseed oil

1/2 large red onion, thinly sliced

3 large shitake mushrooms, thinly sliced

1/2 tsp. grated orange peel

2 c. small broccoli florets

2 small carrots, peeled & julienne cut

1 lb. chicken breast, cut into 3/4" cubes

2 Tbsp. fresh basil, chopped

2 tsp. Bragg's liquid aminos, or to taste

1 tsp. mirin (optional)

> Heat oil in a large skillet over medium heat. Sauté onion, mushrooms and orange peel until lightly browned, about 3-5 minutes.

> Add broccoli and carrots and stir fry an additional 3-5 minutes. Transfer veggies to a bowl and set aside.

> Add more oil to pan if needed and cook chicken for 5 minutes or until done.

> Return veggies to skillet, then season with basil, aminos and mirin. Cook for 1 minute more, or until heated through.

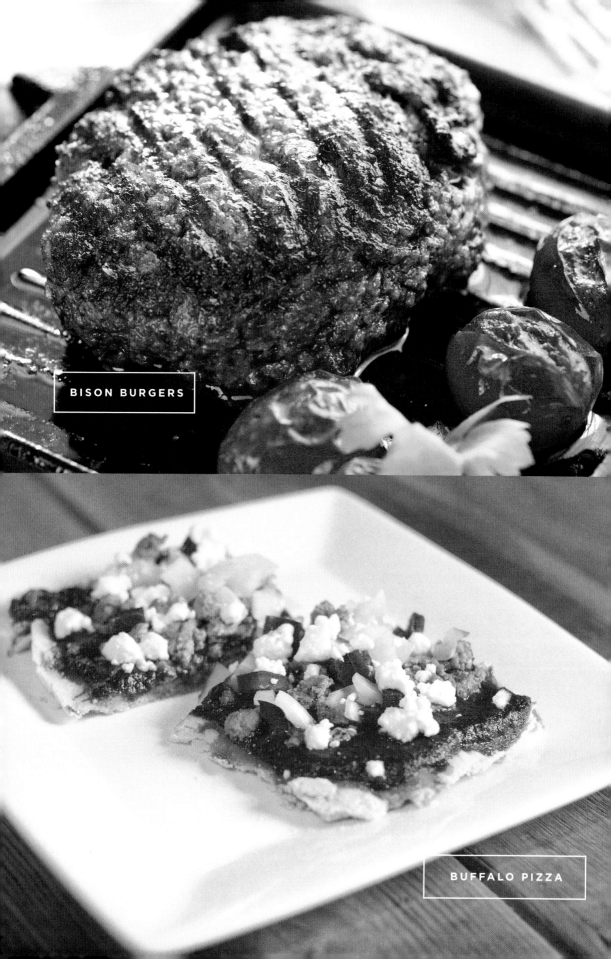

BISON BURGERS

BUFFALO PIZZA

Bison Burgers

2 lbs. ground bison

1 tsp. cumin

1 tsp. onion powder

1 tsp. garlic powder

1 tsp. Bragg's liquid aminos

sea salt & black pepper
to taste

1 Tbsp. coconut oil

> Mix together bison meat and seasonings in a large bowl and form into patties. Heat oil in a large skillet over medium heat and cook patties, flipping once, until done.

> Serve alone, on a bed of greens, or on a sprouted grain bun.

Buffalo Pizza

1 lb. ground bison, browned

1 can organic tomato sauce

1 pkg. crumbled goat cheese

1 red bell pepper, chopped

1 small onion, chopped

Crust:

2 c. brown rice flour

1 tsp. sea salt

1 tsp. stevia

1 Tbsp. grapeseed oil

1 egg

1 c. almond milk

> Mix all crust ingredients in a large bowl. Press into a greased baking dish (9x13) and bake at 425 degrees for 10 minutes.

> Top with sauce, bison, veggies and goat cheese. Reduce oven to 350 degrees and bake for 15 minutes more.

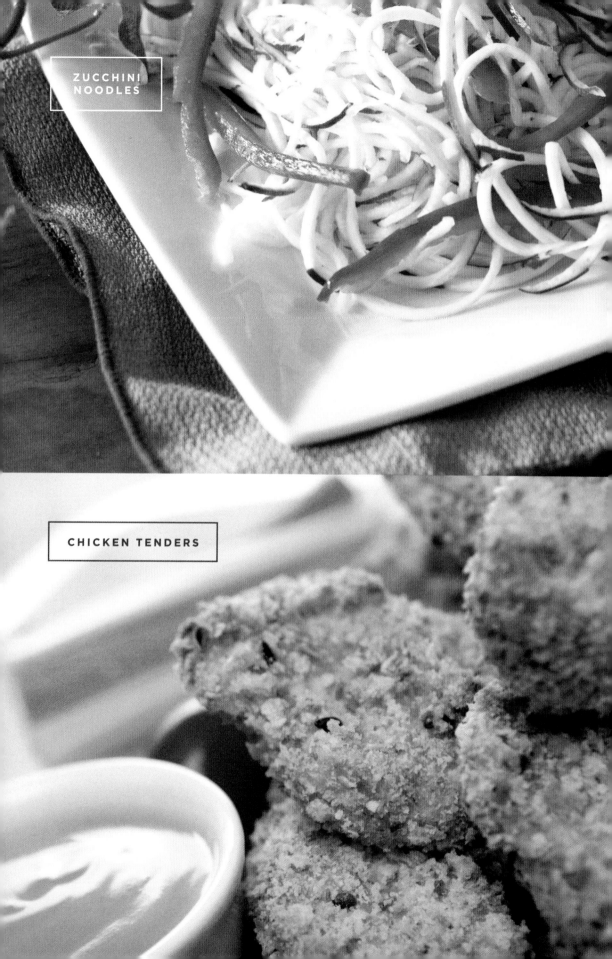

ZUCCHINI
NOODLES

CHICKEN TENDERS

Zucchini Noodles

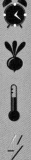

2 c. zucchini, spiralized

1/2 c. red or yellow
bell pepper, thinly sliced

1/4 c. fresh tarragon,
chopped

1 tsp. jalapeno pepper,
minced

1/4 tsp. garlic, minced

2 tsp. ginger, minced

1 Tbsp. lemon juice

1/2 c. shallots, minced

> Combine all ingredients in a bowl
and serve immediately or store in
refrigerator until ready to serve.

Chicken Tenders

2 lbs. chicken breasts,
sliced into strips

2 eggs

Italian seasoning

sea salt

1 c. brown rice or
coconut flour

1 Tbsp. coconut oil

> Beat eggs slightly in a bowl.
Add Italian seasoning and sea salt
to taste. Dip strips of chicken in egg
mixture, then coat with flour.

> Heat coconut oil in a frying pan
over medium heat. Fry chicken,
turning once, until golden brown
and done.

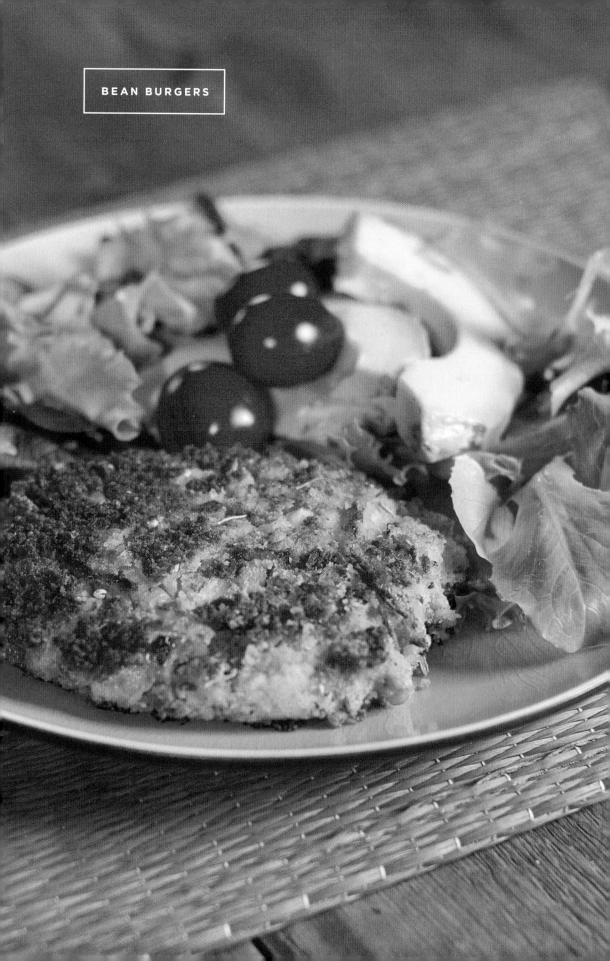

BEAN BURGERS

Bean Burgers

2 c. cooked garbanzo beans

1 1/2 lbs. sweet onion, thinly sliced

2 Tbsp. coconut oil

1/2 c. gluten free breadcrumbs

6 cloves garlic, pressed or minced

2 Tbsp. fresh cilantro, minced

1 Tbsp. fresh rosemary, minced

2 Tbsp. tahini

2 Tbsp. lime juice

1 tsp. sea salt

black pepper to taste

> Heat 1 Tbsp. coconut oil in a large pan and sauté onions until they are soft and begin to caramelize. Season with sea salt and pepper to taste. Place caramelized onions in a large mixing bowl and set aside.

> Place garbanzo beans in a blender or food processor and mix until smooth. Add bean mixture to bowl with onions.

> Add all remaining ingredients and combine thoroughly. Form into patties.

> Heat remaining coconut oil in pan and cook burgers until done, flipping once. Serve with avocado slices and sprouts.

side
dishes

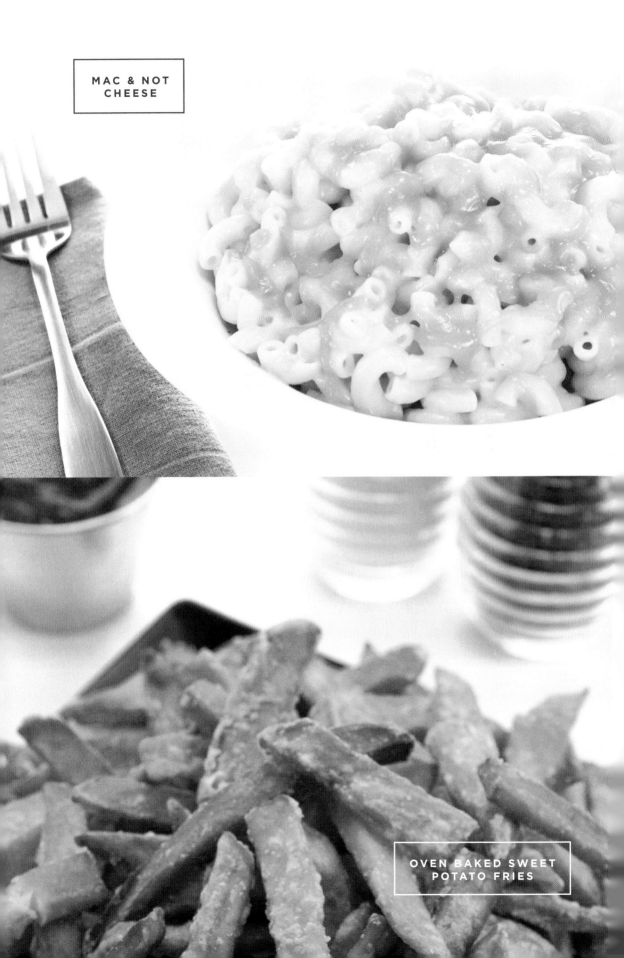

MAC & NOT
CHEESE

OVEN BAKED SWEET
POTATO FRIES

Mac & Not Cheese

1 c. water

1 c. cashews or walnuts

1 Tbsp. sesame seeds

1 1/2 tsp. yeast flakes

1/2 c. pimentos

1/4 tsp. onion powder

1/8 tsp. garlic powder

1/4 c. fresh lemon juice

1/4 c. grapeseed oil

brown rice pasta

> Place 1/2 c. water and all nuts in a blender. Blend then add remaining water.

> Add remaining sauce ingredients and blend well. Pour over warm, cooked pasta.

> Refrigerate any unused sauce.

Oven Baked Sweet Potato Fries

1-1 1/2 lbs. sweet potatoes

1 Tbsp. grapeseed or coconut oil

1/2 tsp. sea salt

1/2 tsp. paprika

1/4 tsp. cinnamon

> Preheat oven to 425 degrees. Peel potatoes and cut into strips about 1/2" wide on each side. Place all ingredients in sealable plastic bag and shake until potatoes are completely coated. Spread onto a baking sheet in a single layer. *For crispier fries, mix non-potato ingredients and lightly brush onto potato slices.

> Cook for 30 minutes, turning every 10 minutes.

> Transfer immediately to a paper towel lined plate and serve warm.

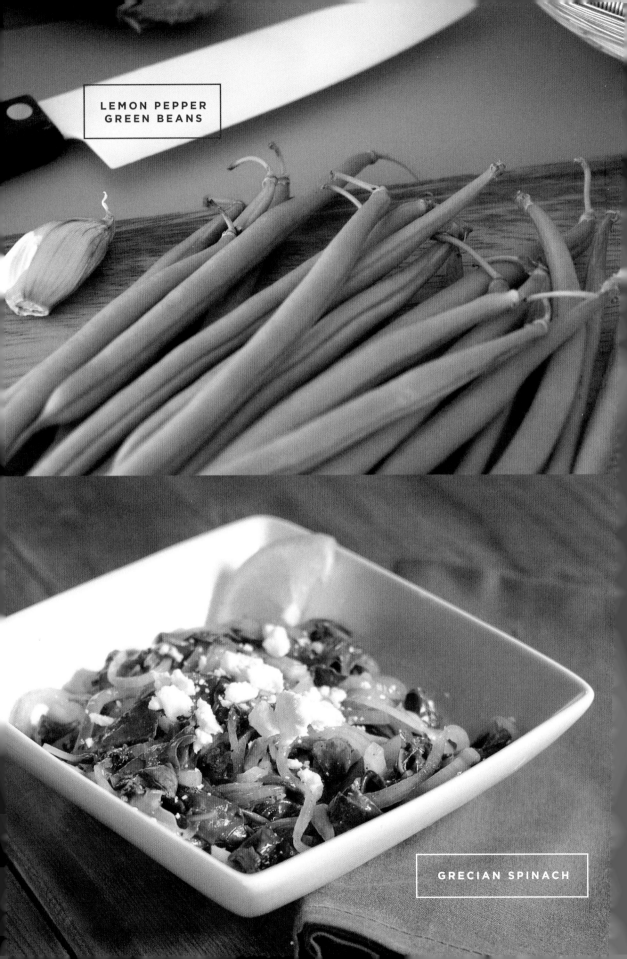

LEMON PEPPER
GREEN BEANS

GRECIAN SPINACH

Lemon Pepper Green Beans

3 lbs. fresh green beans

2 Tbsp. coconut oil or butter

2 cloves garlic, minced

1/4 c. lemon juice

2 tsp. grated lemon zest

sea salt & black pepper
to taste

> Heat oil in a large skillet over medium heat and stir fry green beans and garlic until crisp-tender.

> Reduce heat, add lemon juice, zest, sea salt and pepper.

> Cover and steam for 2-3 minutes, stirring occasionally.

Grecian Spinach

1 Tbsp. coconut oil

1/2 red onion, thinly sliced

16 oz. fresh baby spinach, washed and stemmed

1/2 tsp. grated lemon peel

sea salt & pepper to taste

1/4 c. crumbled feta cheese

> Heat oil in a large skillet over medium heat. Add red onion and sauté 2-3 minutes.

> Add spinach and quickly sauté for 2-3 minutes more.

> Add lemon peel, sea salt and pepper. Cook a few seconds more to release the flavors.

> Stir in feta cheese just prior to serving.

MASHED FAUX-TATOES

BUTTERNUT SQUASH CASSEROLE

Mashed Faux-tatoes

1 med. head cauliflower, abt. 1 1/2 lbs.

1/2 c. raw or organic butter

1/2 tsp. sea salt

5-8 grinds black pepper

minced chives (optional)

> Steam cauliflower until tender.

> In a food processor, blend cauliflower, butter, sea salt and pepper until smooth.

Butternut Squash Casserole

1 small butternut squash, peeled, halved, seeded and thinly sliced

1 small red onion, thinly sliced

1/3 c. unsweetened apple cider or juice

2 Tbsp. grapeseed oil

2 Tbsp. grade B maple syrup

1/4 c. toasted slivered almonds

> Preheat oven to 350 degrees.

> Combine squash and onion in a 9x13 casserole dish. In a small bowl, combine apple cider, oil and syrup. Pour over squash.

> Top with almonds, cover dish with foil and bake for 45 minutes or until tender.

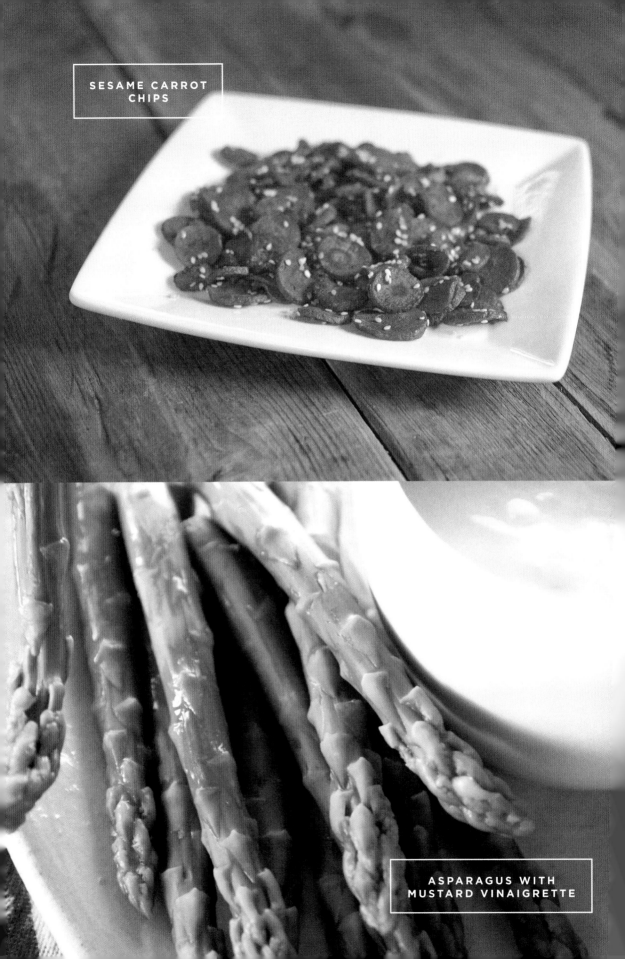

SESAME CARROT CHIPS

ASPARAGUS WITH MUSTARD VINAIGRETTE

Sesame Carrot Chips

2 lbs. carrots, sliced into thin rounds

1 Tbsp. grapeseed oil

1 Tbsp. toasted sesame oil

Sea salt to taste

4 Tbsp. toasted sesame seeds

> Preheat oven to 350 degrees.

> In a large skillet over medium heat, sauté sliced carrots in grapeseed oil until soft (about 6 minutes). Remove from heat and toss with sesame oil and sea salt to taste.

> Spread carrots on a cookie sheet and bake 30 minutes, stirring frequently.

> Remove from oven, toss with sesame seeds and serve warm.

Asparagus with Mustard Vinaigrette

2 lbs. asparagus

3/4 c. pecans

1/2 c. olive oil

1/4 c. red wine vinegar

1 Tbsp. stoneground mustard

1/8 tsp. sea salt

freshly ground black pepper

> Preheat oven to 300 degrees.

> Whisk together olive oil, red wine vinegar, mustard and spices in a small bowl and set aside.

> Place pecans on a cookie sheet and toast until fragrant and lightly browned. Remove and set aside to cool.

> Discard tough ends of asparagus and steam asparagus until it turns bright green (about 3 minutes). Remove from heat and place on serving dish. Drizzle with vinaigrette, top with pecans and serve immediately.

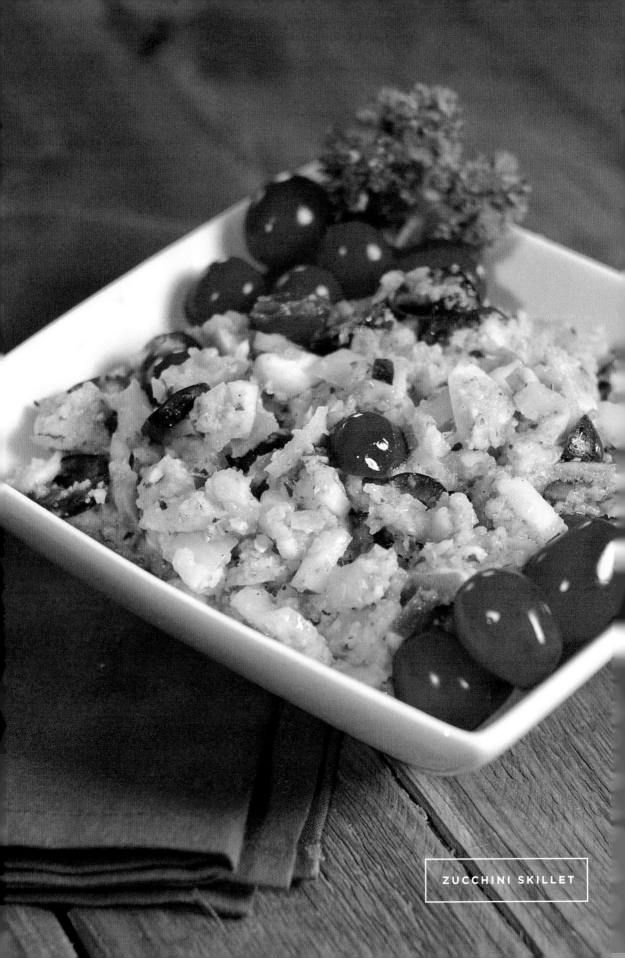

ZUCCHINI SKILLET

Turnip Fries

4 turnips, cut into steak fries

1 Tbsp. grapeseed oil

1/2 tsp. garlic powder

sea salt & black pepper to taste

> Preheat oven to 425 degrees.

> In a large bowl, toss all ingredients until turnip fries are well coated. Place in a single layer on a cookie sheet and bake 15-20 minutes.

> Flip fries and bake for an additional 15-20 minutes.

Zucchini Skillet

1/2 c. chopped onion

3 Tbsp. grapeseed oil

3 c. coarsely shredded zucchini

2 tsp. minced fresh basil

1/2 tsp. sea salt

1/8 tsp. garlic powder

1 c. diced fresh tomatoes

2 Tbsp. sliced, ripe black olives

> Heat oil in a large skillet over medium heat. Sauté onions, zucchini, basil, sea salt and garlic powder for 5-6 minutes.

> Sprinkle with tomatoes and olives. Cover and cook for 5 more minutes.

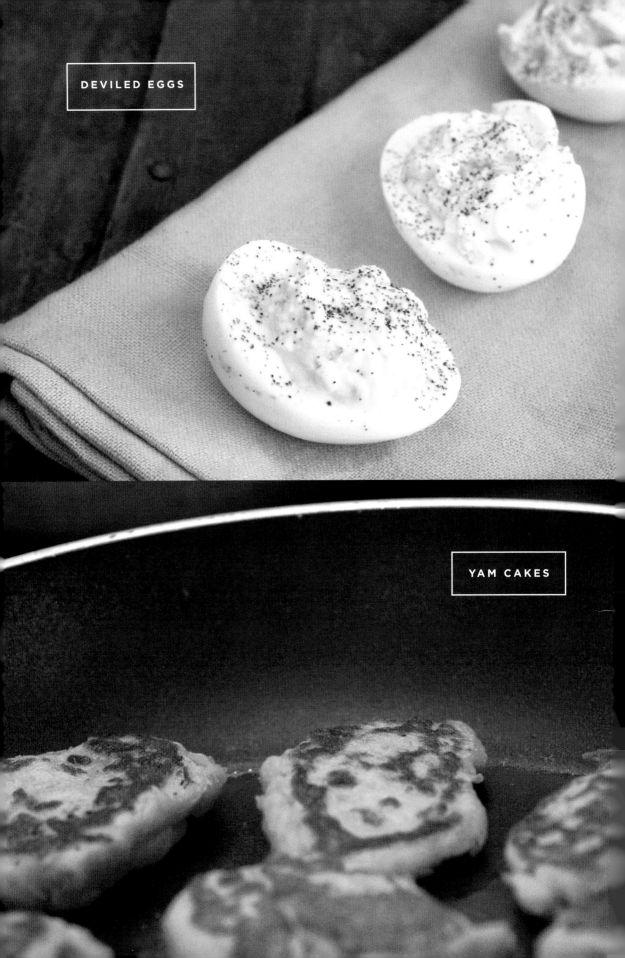

DEVILED EGGS

YAM CAKES

Deviled Eggs

10 cage-free eggs

1 c. mayonnaise alternative (like Veganaise w/ grapeseed oil)

1/4 c. organic mustard

1/2 tsp. apple cider vinegar

paprika

> Hard boil eggs in a sauce pan of boiling water for 20 minutes. Let eggs cool, peel, then cut in half and remove yolks.

> Mix yolks with Veganaise, mustard and apple cider vinegar. Spoon yolk mixture into egg white halves.

> Sprinkle with paprika on top.

Yam Cakes

1-2 yams or sweet potatoes

1 c. almond or coconut milk

cinnamon to taste

1 Tbsp. coconut oil

berries (optional)

maple syrup (optional)

> Poke holes in the yam or sweet potato with a fork and place on a baking sheet. Cook at 400 degrees for 45-50 minutes or until soft.

> Use food processor or blender to mix cooked yams or sweet potatoes with cinnamon and any additional seasonings.

> Place yam mixture in a large bowl and add milk until desired consistency is reached (as with any pancake mix).

> Heat coconut oil in skillet over medium heat. Drop batter into skillet and cook 2-3 minutes on each side, or until golden brown.

> Top with cinnamon, berries or a small amount of maple syrup.

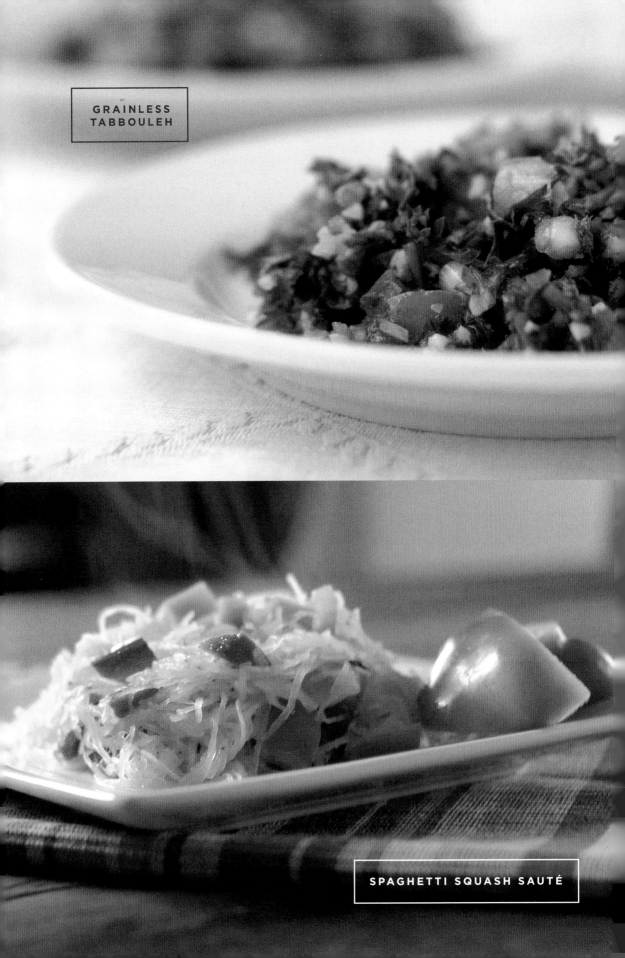

GRAINLESS
TABBOULEH

SPAGHETTI SQUASH SAUTÉ

Grainless Tabbouleh

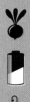

2 c. curly parsley, chopped

2 c. flat-leaf Italian parsley, chopped

2 med. cucumbers, peeled, seeded, finely diced

3/4 c. finely chopped tomatoes

3/4 c. finely diced celery

1 c. chopped fresh mint leaves

1 Tbsp. pine nuts

2 Tbsp. fresh lemon juice

2 Tbsp. olive oil

1 tsp. sea salt

3 grinds fresh black pepper

> Combine parsley, cucumber, tomatoes, celery, mint leaves and pine nuts in a medium bowl and set aside.

> Mix lemon juice, olive oil, sea salt and pepper in a separate bowl. Pour mixture over salad and toss well to mix.

> Serve immediately.

Spaghetti Squash Sauté

1 large spaghetti squash

2 Tbsp. raw or organic butter

1 med. shallot, minced

2 Tbsp. red pepper, finely chopped

2 Tbsp. green pepper, finely chopped

1/2 tsp. Italian seasoning

fresh ground pepper to taste

> Cut squash in half and boil in a large pot filled with water until tender. Remove from pot and allow to cool slightly. Scoop out flesh with a fork.

> In a large skillet, melt butter over medium heat and sauté shallot for about a minute.

> Add squash, peppers and seasoning and stir to mix. Cook until dish is heated through, about 2-3 minutes.

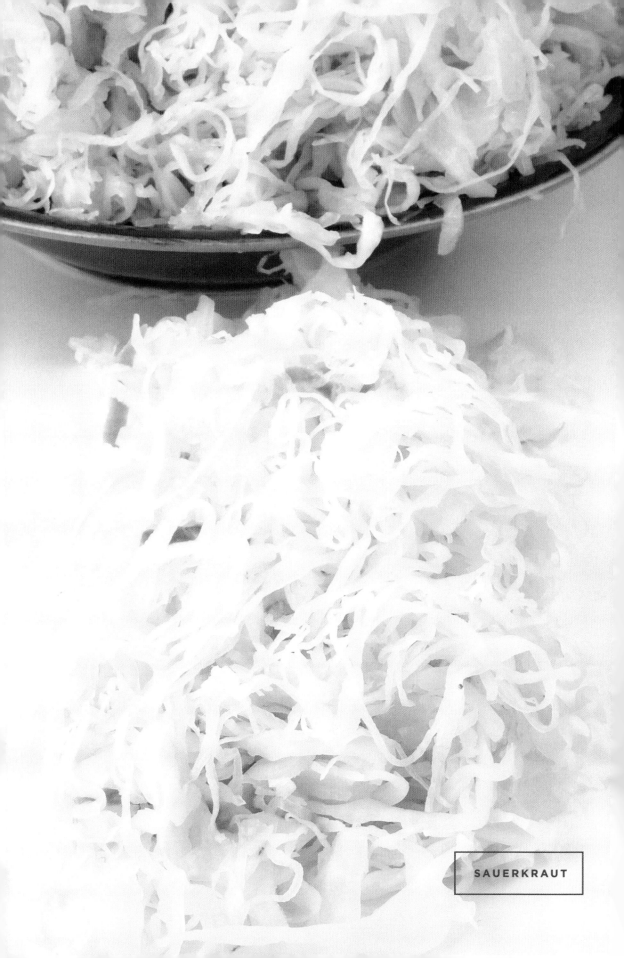

SAUERKRAUT

Sauerkraut

2 lbs. shredded green cabbage (abt 2 qts., loosely packed)

2 Tbsp. sea salt

1 tsp. caraway or cumin seeds

2 c. filtered water

> Slice cabbage thinly and place in a large bowl. Mash or pound cabbage with a heavy cup, pestle or mallet until cabbage starts to release juice.

> Sprinkle with seeds and mix well. Place mixture into 2 quart mason jars.

> Stir sea salt into water and pour over cabbage to within 3/4" from the top of the jar.

> Replace lid and store at room temperature for 3 days, then place in refrigerator.

snacks

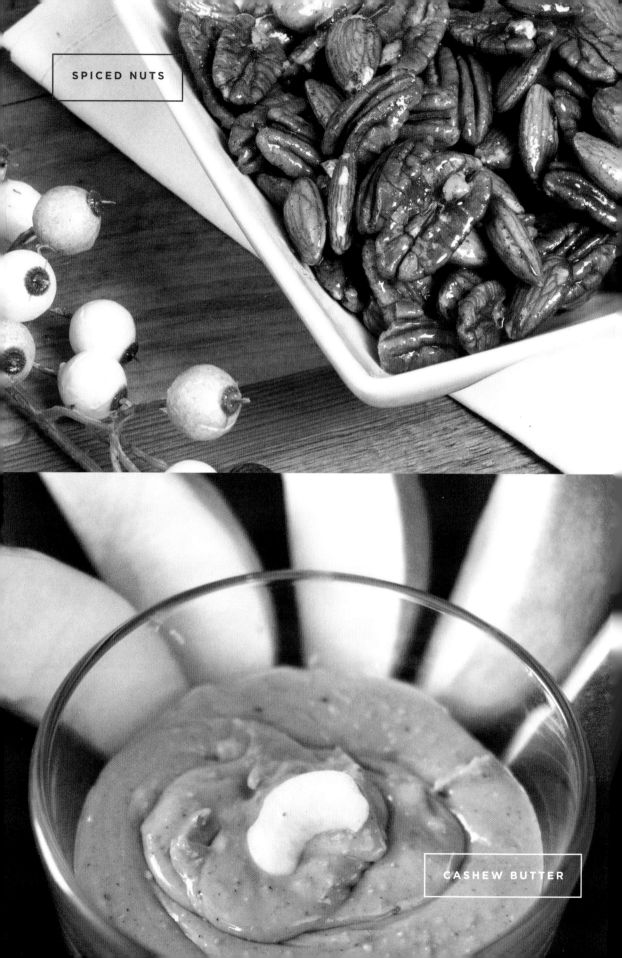

SPICED NUTS

CASHEW BUTTER

Spiced Nuts

1/2 c. honey

1-2 c. pecans, almonds or walnuts

1 tsp. cinnamon

1/4 tsp. cayenne pepper (optional)

> Combine all ingredients in a bowl and toss until nuts are completely coated.

> Spread nuts on a cookie sheet in a single layer and toast at 300 degrees, tossing occasionally, until fragrant, about 4-5 minutes.

> Serve on top of a salad or eat by themselves.

Cashew Butter

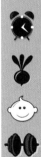

1/4 c. sesame oil or grapeseed oil

1/4 lb. raw cashew pieces

1-2 dates (optional)

sea salt to taste

> Pour oil into blender. Add cashew pieces and blend until desired consistency is reached.

> Add 1-2 dates if desired and blend once more.

> Serve as a dip for apple slices, veggies, etc. or use in other recipes.

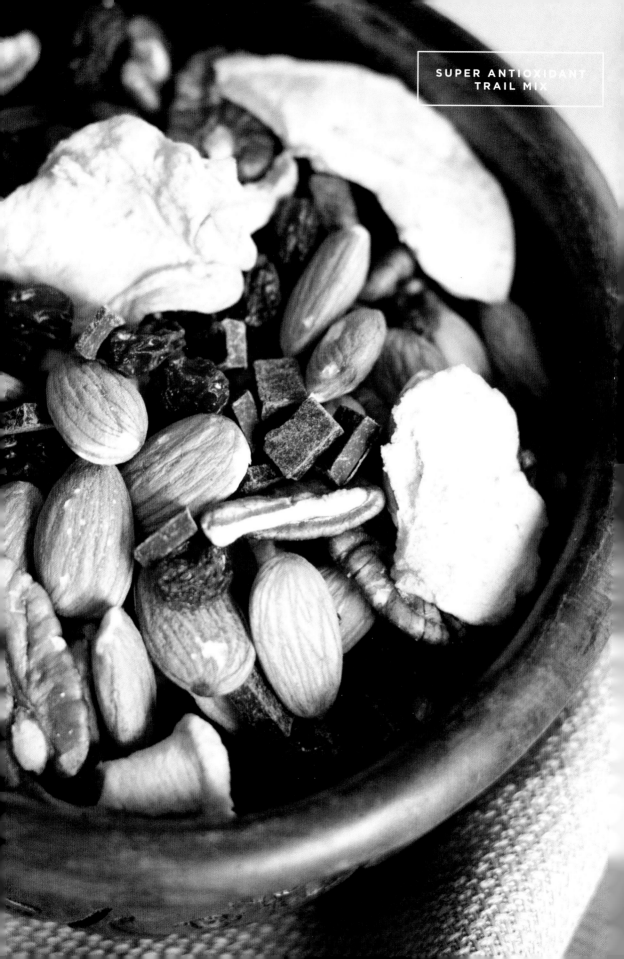

Super Antioxidant Trail Mix

1 c. pecans

1 c. almonds

1/2 c. raisins

1/2 c. dark chocolate chips (unsweetened)

1 c. dried apple slices

sea salt & cinnamon to taste

> Mix all ingredients together in a bowl.

Blueberry Bliss Snack Bar

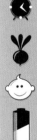

1/4 c. dried blueberries

1/4 c. dates

1/3 c. almonds

1/2 tsp. finely grated lemon zest

1 drop almond extract

> Place dates, dried blueberries, lemon zest and almond extract in a food processor and blend to a paste. Set aside in a bowl.

> Place nuts in food processor and pulse until finely chopped.

> Add nuts to bowl and knead together with fingers and form into bars. Store in refrigerator.

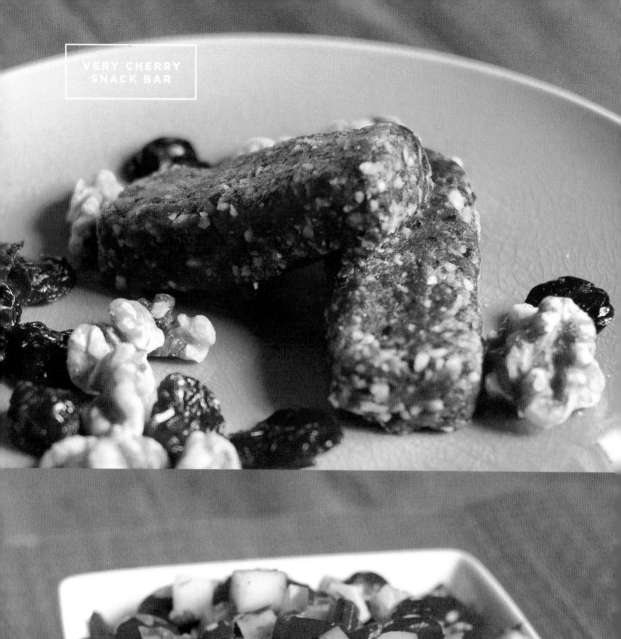

VERY CHERRY
SNACK BAR

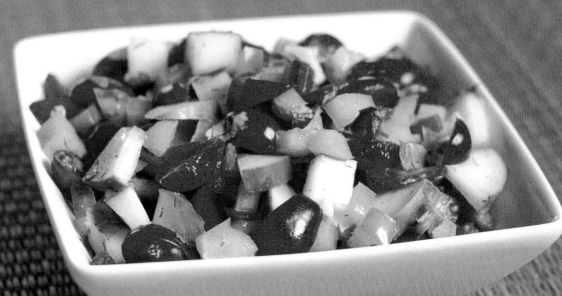

CUCUMBER SALSA

Very Cherry Snack Bar

1/4 c. dates

1/4 c. dried cherries

1/3 c. pecans, almonds or walnuts

1/8 tsp. cinnamon

> Place dates, dried cherries and cinnamon in a food processor and blend to a paste. Set aside in a bowl.

> Place nuts in food processor and pulse until finely chopped.

> Add nuts to bowl and knead together with fingers and form into bars. Store in refrigerator.

Cucumber Salsa

3 c. cherry tomatoes, quartered

1 c. green, red & yellow peppers, chopped

2 med. cucumbers, peeled, seeded & chopped

1 jalapeno pepper, seeded & chopped

1 sm. Vidalia onion

1 clove garlic, minced

4 Tbsp. lime juice

1 tsp. fresh parsley, minced

> Mix all ingredients together in a large bowl.

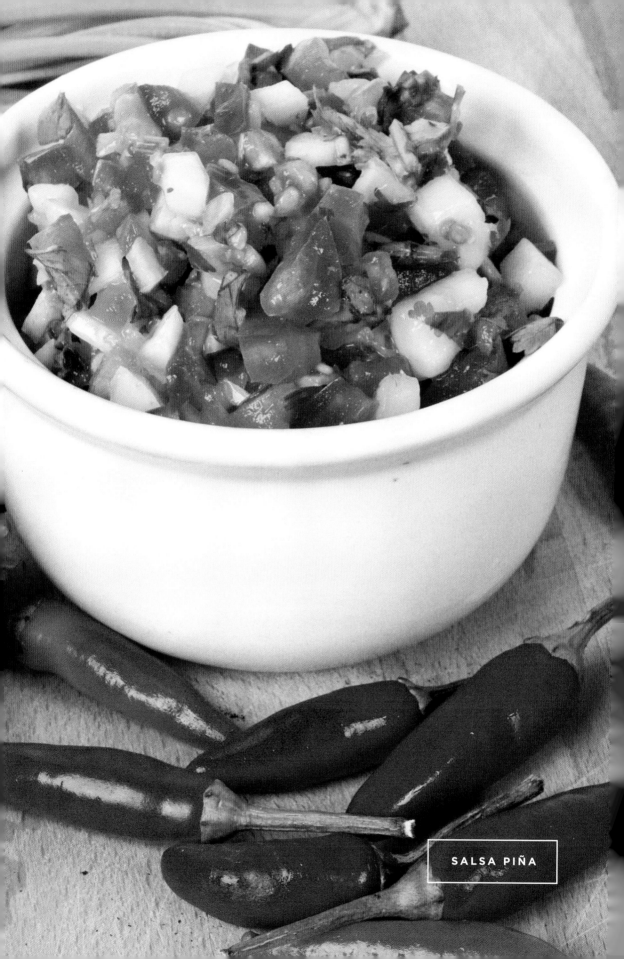

SALSA PIÑA

Salsa Piña

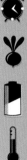

1 1/2 c. fresh pineapple, chopped

1 c. cherry tomatoes, quartered

1/4 c. Vidalia onion, chopped

1/4 c. red onion, chopped

1/4 c. red bell pepper, chopped

2 fresh chili peppers, seeded

2-3 Tbsp. fresh lime juice

1/4 tsp. sea salt

1 Tbsp. olive oil

1/4 c. fresh cilantro, chopped

> Mix all ingredients together in a large bowl.

Fruit Salsa

2 kiwis, peeled & diced

2 apples, peeled, cored & diced

8 oz. raspberries

1 lb. strawberries

1 Tbsp. stevia

3 Tbsp. organic fruit preserves

> Mix all ingredients together in a large bowl.

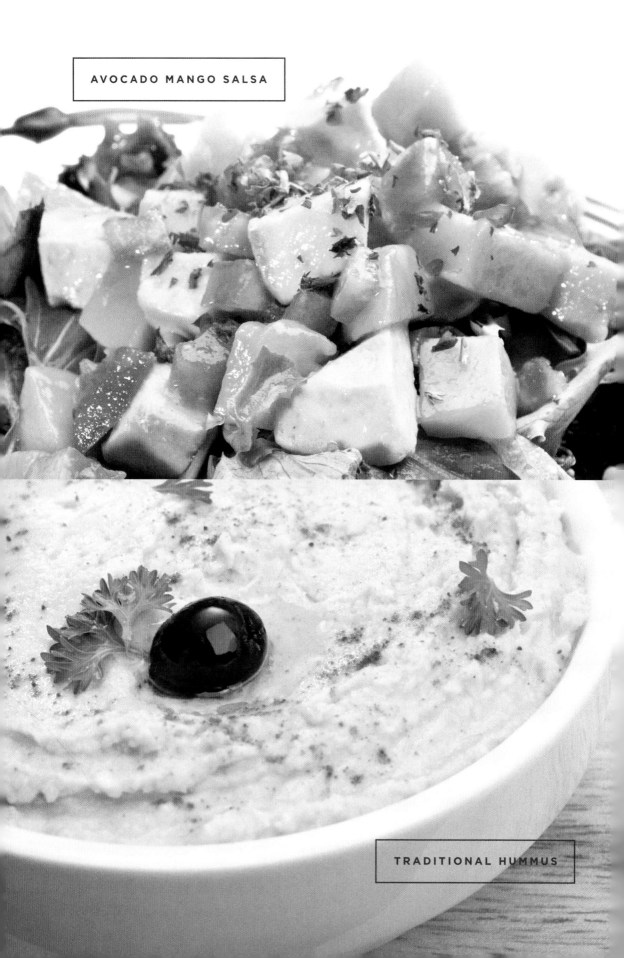

AVOCADO MANGO SALSA

TRADITIONAL HUMMUS

Avocado Mango Salsa

1 mango, peeled, seeded & diced

1 avocado, peeled, pitted & diced

4 medium tomatoes, diced

1 jalapeno pepper, seeded & minced

1/2 c. fresh cilantro

3 cloves garlic, minced

1 tsp. sea salt

2 Tbsp. fresh lime juice

1/4 c. chopped red onion

3 Tbsp. olive oil

> Mix all ingredients together in a large bowl.

Traditional Hummus

2 cans garbanzo beans

1/4 c. raw sesame seeds

1 Tbsp. olive oil

1/4 c. lemon juice

1 garlic clove, peeled

1 tsp. cumin

sea salt to taste

> Drain and rinse garbanzo beans, reserving 1/4 c. liquid.

> Place all ingredients in a blender and blend. Add more water or olive oil until desired consistency is reached.

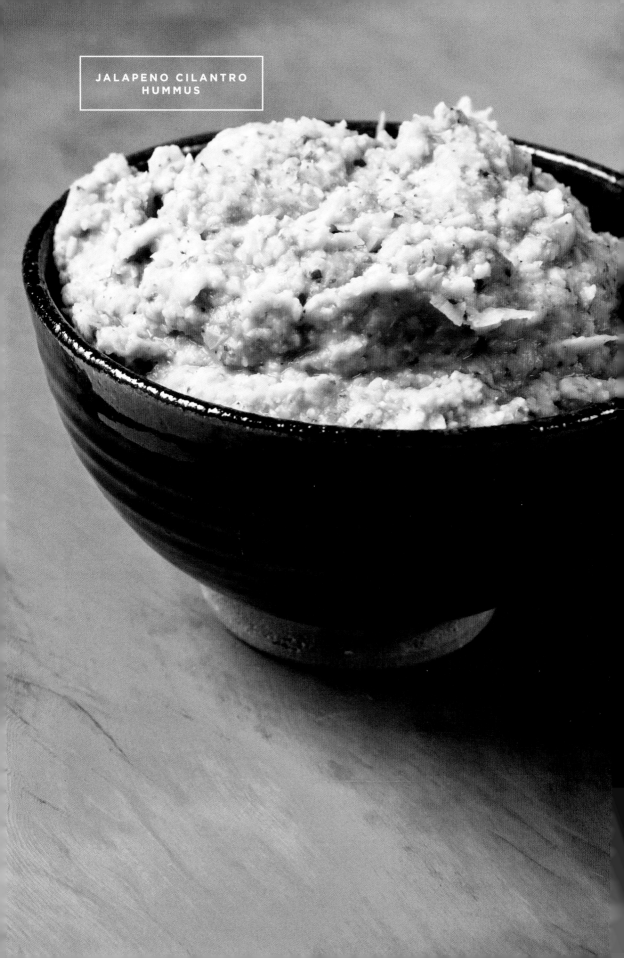

JALAPENO CILANTRO
HUMMUS

Black Bean Hummus

1 can garbanzo beans

1 can black beans

1/3 c. tahini

6 cloves garlic, peeled

4 Tbsp. olive oil

2 Tbsp. lemon juice

1 tsp. sea salt

> Blend ingredients in a blender or food processor.

> Use as a spread or dip with bell pepper slices, carrot sticks or celery.

Jalapeno Cilantro Hummus

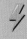

2 cloves garlic

2 cans garbanzo beans

3 Tbsp. lime juice

1/2 tsp. sea salt

1/2 c. olive oil

3/4 c. fresh cilantro, chopped

2 jalapeno peppers, seeded & minced

> Place all ingredients in a food processor or blender and blend together.

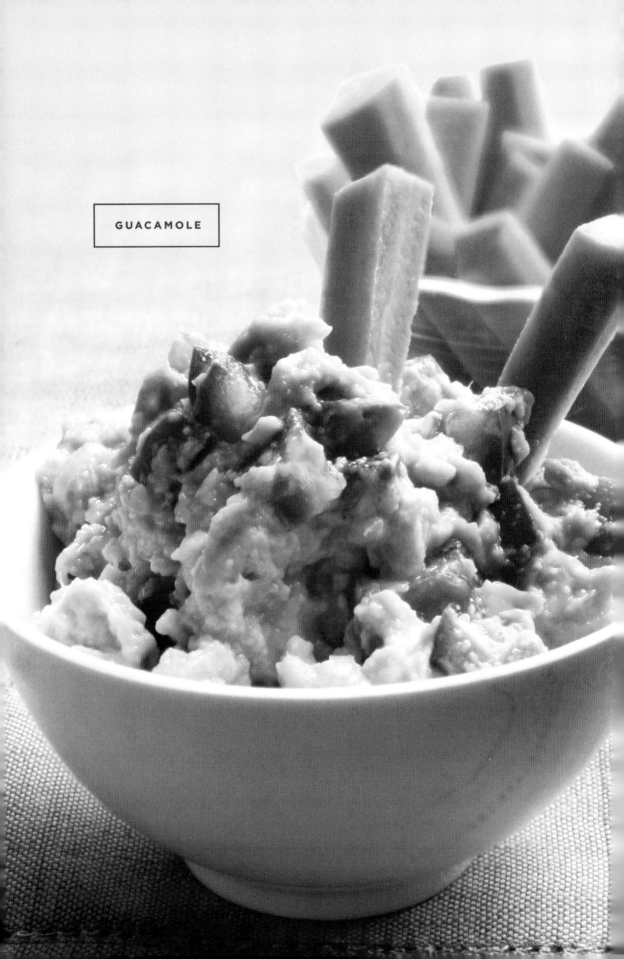

GUACAMOLE

Guacamole

2 avocados

1 lime

2 cloves garlic, minced

1 small tomato or salsa

1 tsp. sea salt

1/2 tsp. dill

> Spoon out avocado into a large bowl. Add lime juice, minced garlic and chopped tomato. Mash together until mixture becomes creamy.

> Add sea salt and dill.

> Refrigerate and serve with bell pepper slices, celery or carrots.

Veggie Dip

1 c. mayonnaise alternative (like Vegenaise with grapeseed oil)

2 Tbsp. organic mustard

1/4 c. oil & vinegar dressing (see pg 121)

> Combine all ingredients in a bowl and mix well.

Perfect for veggie trays to take to parties.

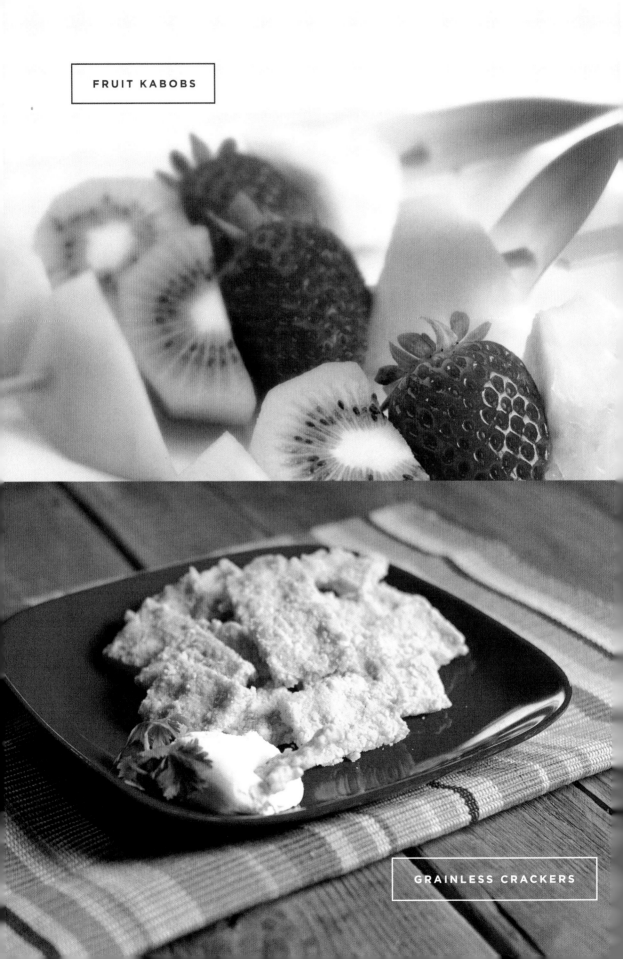

FRUIT KABOBS

GRAINLESS CRACKERS

Fruit Kabobs

pieces of fruit
(such as red or green grapes,
blueberries, strawberries,
raspberries, apple cut into
cubes, etc.)

raw cheddar cheese,
cut into cubes

toothpicks or kabob sticks

> Slide fruit and cheese on
toothpicks or kabob sticks.

Grainless Crackers

3 c. almond flour

1 1/2 tsp. Celtic sea salt

1 c. sesame seeds

2 eggs, whisked until frothy

2 Tbsp. grapeseed oil

> Stir together all ingredients in a
large mixing bowl until well combined.
Separate dough into two halves.

> Line 2 large baking sheets with
parchment paper. Place one half of
the dough on each baking sheet. With
another layer of parchment paper
over the top of the dough, roll out the
dough until it is about 1/8 inch thick
and covers the whole baking sheet.

> Repeat with the other half of
the dough.

> Remove the top layer of parchment
paper and cut dough into 2 inch
squares with a knife or pizza cutter.

> Bake at 350 degrees for 10-12
minutes or until golden brown.

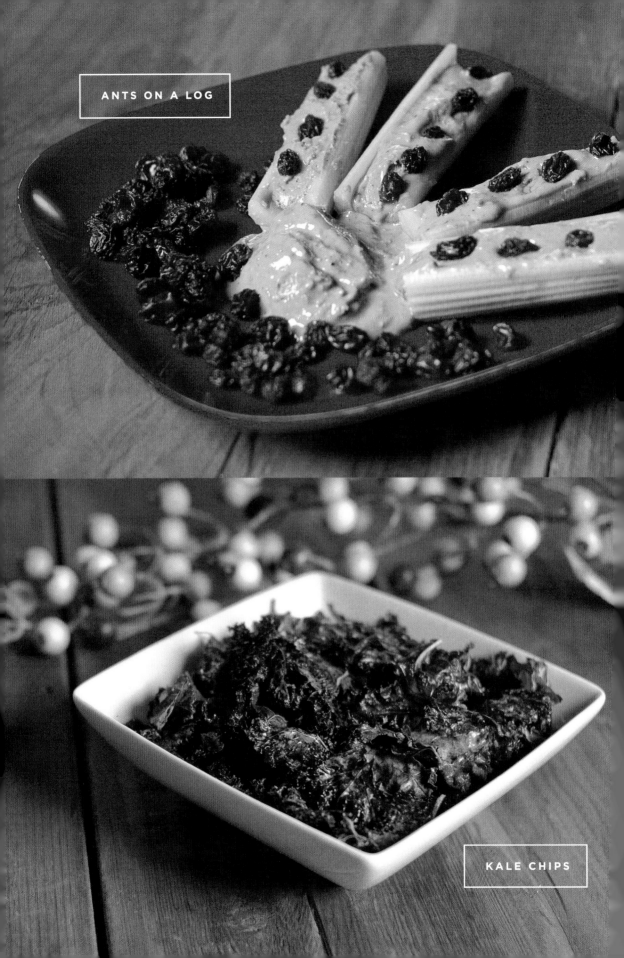

ANTS ON A LOG

KALE CHIPS

Ants on a Log

1 bunch celery

1 c. cashew or
almond butter

1/4 c. raisins

> Spread nut butter into individual
celery stalks and top with raisins.

Kale Chips

1 bunch kale

2 Tbsp. grapeseed oil

1 Tbsp. lemon juice

1/4 tsp. sea salt

> Preheat oven to 350 degrees.

> Chop kale into 1/2 inch pieces.

> Place all ingredients in a large
bowl and massage the oil, lemon
juice and sea salt into the kale using
your hands.

> Place on parchment lined baking
sheets and bake for 12 minutes.

desserts

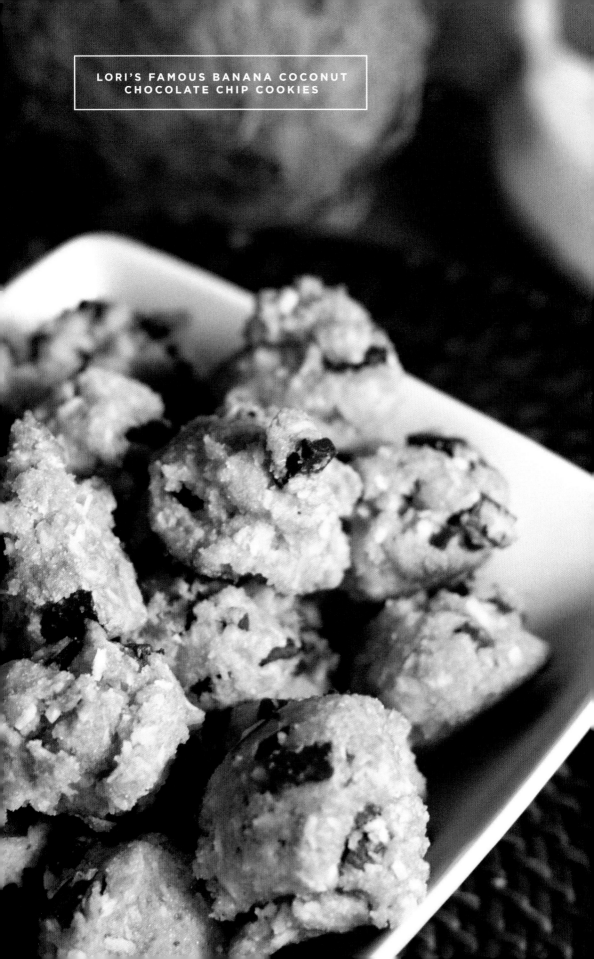

Lori's Famous Banana Coconut Chocolate Chip Cookies

2 bananas

1/4 c. grapeseed oil

1/4 c. grade B maple syrup

1/2 tsp. vanilla extract

2/3 c. flax meal

1 c. brown rice flour

1/4 tsp. baking soda

1/2 c. shredded, unsweetened coconut flakes

pinch of sea salt

1/4 c. dark chocolate chips

> Preheat oven to 350 degrees.

> Combine bananas, oil, syrup and vanilla in a medium bowl or blender. In a separate bowl, combine flours, coconut, baking soda and salt. Add banana mixture to dry ingredients and blend until just combined. Fold in chocolate chips.

> Drop batter onto cookie sheet by heaping teaspoons. Bake 14 minutes or until golden brown.

> Place on wire rack to cool.

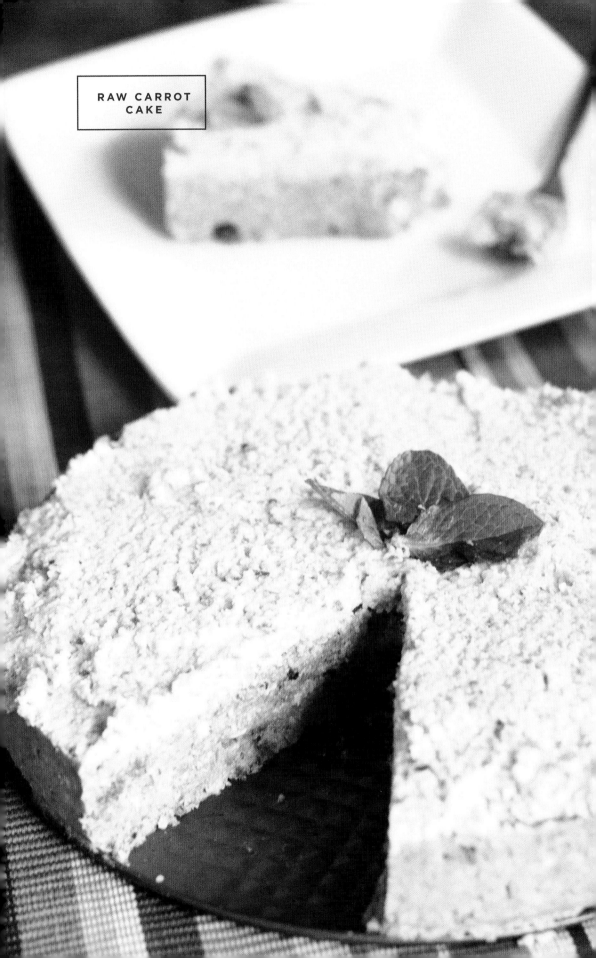

RAW CARROT
CAKE

Raw Carrot Cake

1/2 lb. carrots

1 c. pineapple

1 apple

1 c. soaked almonds

1 1/4 c. soaked walnuts

1 1/4 c. pecans

1 c. pumpkin seeds

1/2 tsp. cinnamon

1/2 c. dates

1/2 c. raisins

1 tsp. pumpkin pie spice

1 1/2 Tbsp. psyllium powder

> Place half the raisins and all of the dates in a food processor or powerful blender and mix to a paste.

> Add soaked almonds and mix in blender. Then add 1 c. walnuts, 1 c. pecans, pumpkin seeds and spices and mix again. Place mixture in a bowl.

> Place remaining 1/4 c. walnuts and 1/4 c. pecans in the food processor and mix into small chucks. Add to dough in bowl.

> Chop carrots and mix in food processor or powerful blender. Add pineapple, apple and psyllium powder and mix together.

> Add carrot mixture to dough and combine well by hand. Pour dough into a springform pan.

Frosting:

3/4 c. soaked and blanched almonds

1/2 c. dates

1/4 tsp. cinnamon

1 pinch clove

1/2 Thai coconut (also called Jelly coconut)

> Place dates, blanched almonds, coconut meat & juice, cinnamon and clove into a blender. Mix until it forms a cream. Spread over the cake.

> Chill cake in the refrigerator for at least 2 hours before serving.

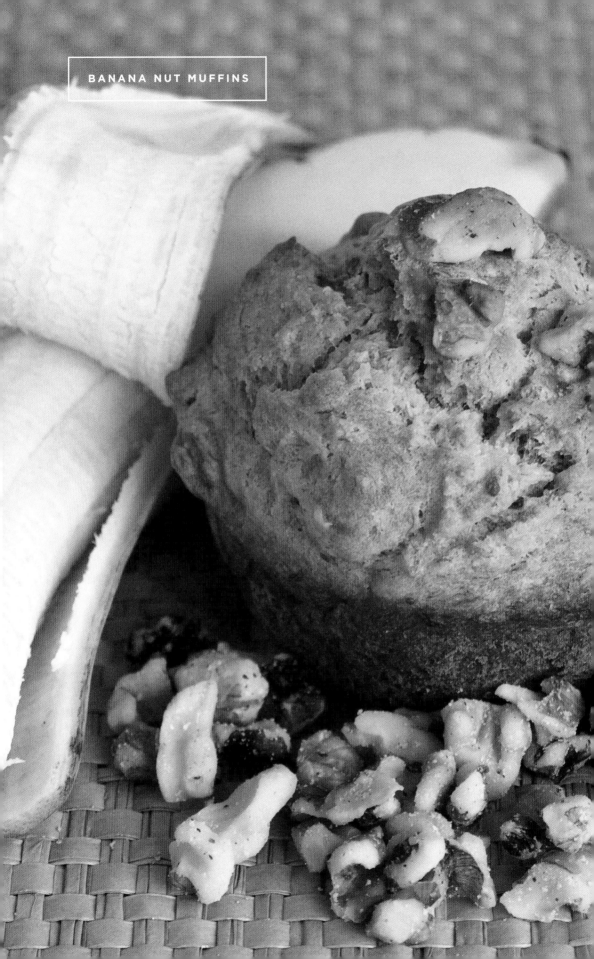

Banana Nut Muffins

1 3/4 c. gluten free flour

2/3 c. maple syrup or honey

1 tsp. baking powder

1 tsp. baking soda

1/2 tsp. sea salt

1 egg

1/2 c. grapeseed oil

1/2 c. goat's milk yogurt
or coconut milk

1 tsp. vanilla extract

1 c. mashed ripe bananas

3/4 c. dark chocolate chips

1/2 c. pecans or walnuts

> In a large bowl, combine flour, baking powder, baking soda and sea salt.

> In a separate bowl, combine maple syrup, egg, oil, yogurt and vanilla.

> Stir wet ingredients into dry until just moistened. Fold in bananas, chocolate chips and nuts.

> Fill greased or paper-lined muffin cups 2/3 full. Bake at 350 degrees for 22-25 minutes or until a toothpick comes out clean.

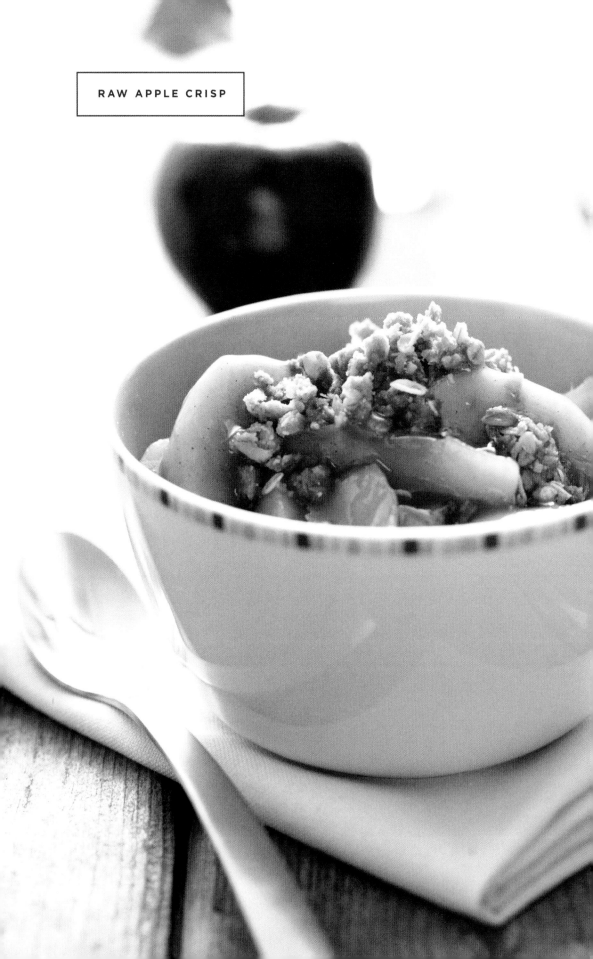

RAW APPLE CRISP

Raw Apple Crisp

8 apples, peeled & chopped

1 c. raisins, soaked & drained

2 tsp. cinnamon, divided

1/4 tsp. nutmeg

2 Tbsp. lemon juice

2 c. walnuts

1 c. pitted dates

1/8 tsp. sea salt

> Place 2 apples, raisins, 1 tsp. cinnamon & nutmeg in a food processor and process until smooth.

> Toss remaining chopped apples with lemon juice in a large bowl. Pour apple raisin puree over apples and mix well.

> Spoon mixture into a medium sized baking dish and set aside.

Crumble:

> Pulse walnuts, dates, 1 tsp. cinnamon and sea salt in a food processor until coarsely ground. Be careful not to over mix.

> Sprinkle mixture over apples and press down lightly with your hands.

> Serve immediately or let sit for a few hours for the flavor to marinate.

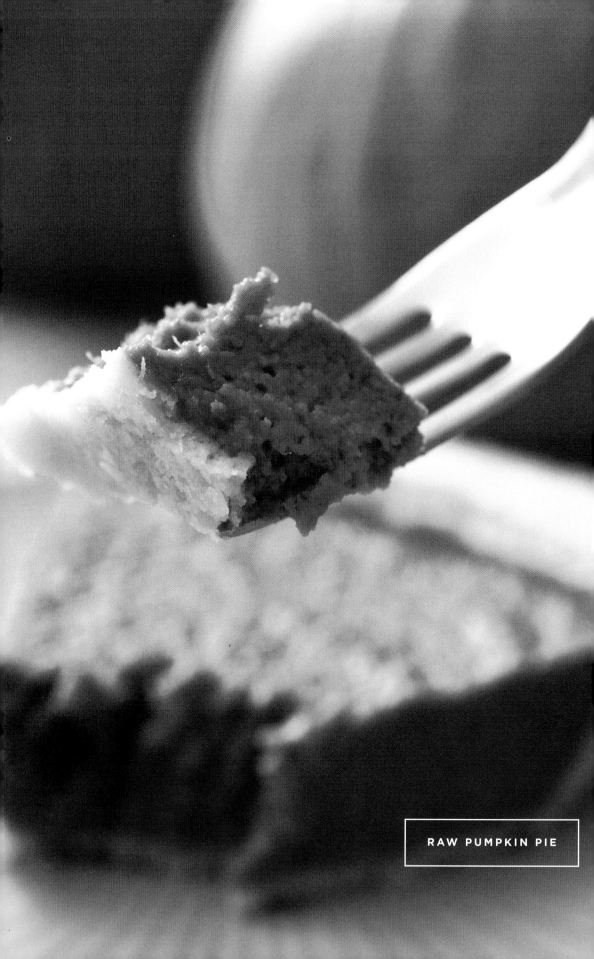

RAW PUMPKIN PIE

Raw Pumpkin Pie

Crust:

2 c. pecans or walnuts

1/2 c. soaked dates

dash sea salt

> Blend the crust ingredients in a powerful blender or food processor.

> Evenly distribute in the bottom of a pie plate, pressing down gently with your fingers.

Filling:

2 c. shredded pumpkin, butternut squash or sweet potato flesh

1 c. soaked dates

2 tsp. cinnamon

1 tsp. freshly diced ginger

1 tsp. nutmeg

1 tsp. coconut oil

dash vanilla

1/4 c. almond milk or water to help blend

> Mix all ingredients together in a blender. Pour into crust.

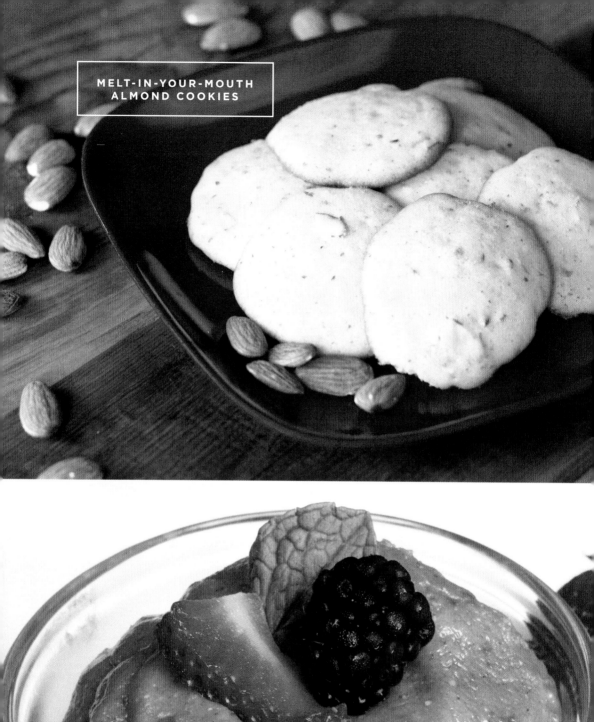

MELT-IN-YOUR-MOUTH
ALMOND COOKIES

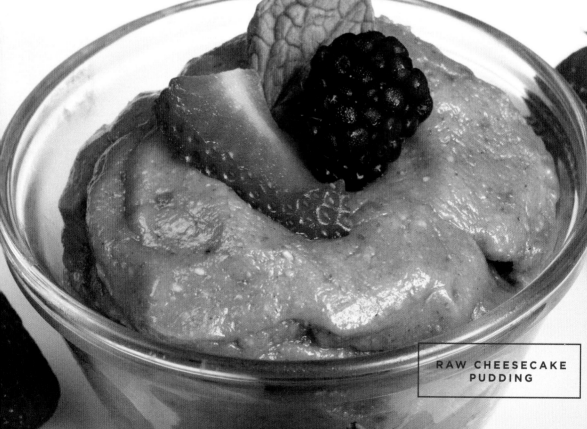

RAW CHEESECAKE
PUDDING

Melt-in-Your-Mouth Almond Cookies

1/2 c. organic butter

1 egg

1/3 c. honey

1 Tbsp. coconut milk

1/2 tsp. almond extract

3/4 c. gluten free flour

3/4 c. coconut flour

1/4 tsp. sea salt

1/4 tsp. baking soda

1/2 c. slivered almonds

> Cream the butter, egg, honey, coconut milk and almond extract in a large bowl until thoroughly combined. Add flours, sea salt, baking soda and almonds. Mix together well.

> Drop batter onto cookie sheet by the teaspoon. Bake at 350 degrees for 12-15 minutes or until golden brown.

Raw Cheesecake Pudding

1 c. raw cashew butter (see pg 187)

1/3 c. lemon juice

1/3 c. raw honey

4 dates

1 tsp. vanilla

1/2 tsp. Celtic sea salt

> Blend all ingredients until smooth.

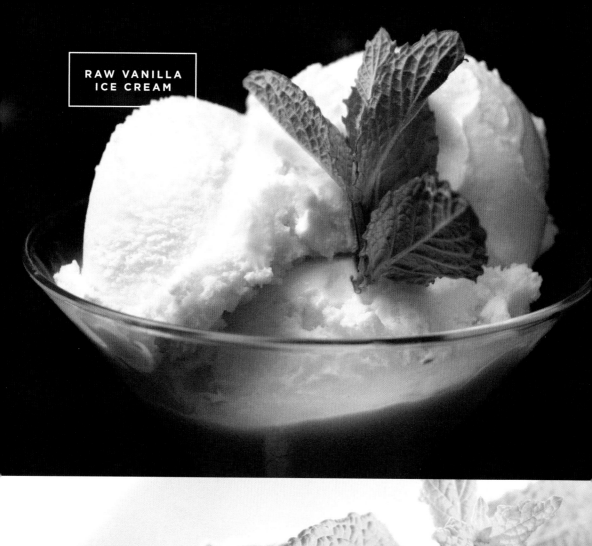

RAW VANILLA
ICE CREAM

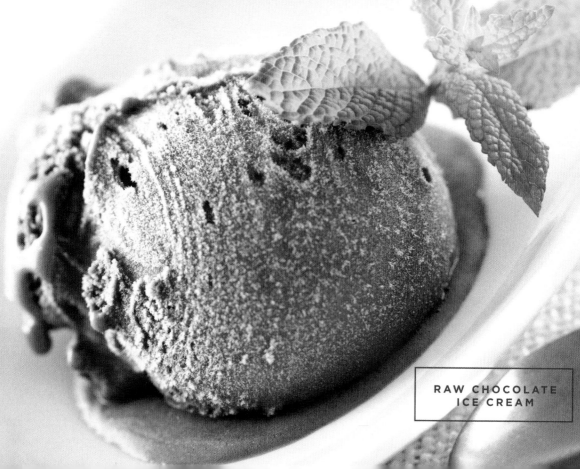

RAW CHOCOLATE
ICE CREAM

Raw Vanilla Ice Cream

Meat of 3 young coconuts

1 Tbsp. pure vanilla beans

1/2 c. pure maple syrup

4 c. ice cubes (abt. 14 cubes)

> Place coconut meat, vanilla beans, maple syrup and 1 c. ice cubes in a high powered blender and blend until desired consistency is reached, adding the remaining ice cubes gradually.

> Add coconut water if mixture is too thick.

Raw Chocolate Ice Cream

3 bananas

3 Tbsp. unsweetened dark cocoa powder

2 Tbsp. raw, unsalted tahini

8 packets stevia

6 organic dates, pitted

3-4 c. ice cubes

> Place bananas, cocoa powder, tahini, stevia, dates and 1 c. ice in a high powered blender and blend until desired consistency is reached, adding remaining ice cubes gradually.

> Add coconut water if mixture is too thick.

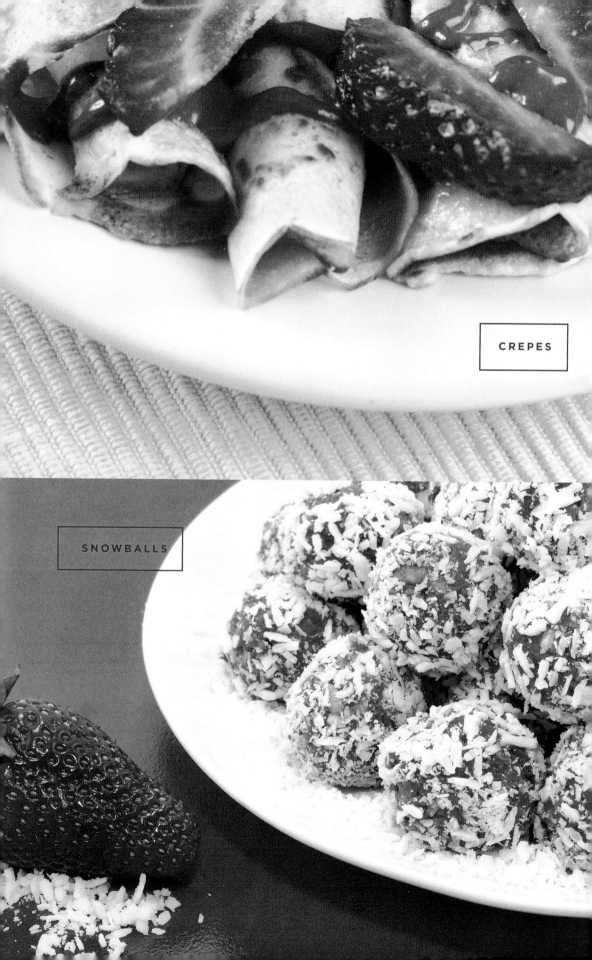

CREPES

SNOWBALLS

Crepes

2 large eggs

1 c. coconut milk

1/2 c. water

1/4 tsp. sea salt

1/2 tsp. vanilla extract

1/2 tsp. grated nutmeg

1 c. garbanzo bean flour

2 Tbsp. organic butter
or coconut oil

> Place eggs, milk, water, sea salt, nutmeg, vanilla, flour and butter or oil in a blender and blend on a medium setting for about 10 seconds, or until just mixed.

> Let batter rest for 30 minutes to 1 hour.

> Heat a skillet over medium heat until hot. Grease with a small amount of grapeseed or coconut oil, then pour 1/4 c. of batter into pan, rotating pan to distribute batter evenly. Cook 1-2 minutes, or until crepe is golden on the bottom.

> Flip with a spatula and cook less than a minute on opposite side. Repeat until all batter has been used.

> Use as a wrap for meat and/or veggies or fill with dessert-like fillings such as berries and chocolate fondue sauce (see page 225)

Snowballs

1 c. almond butter

2 Tbsp. raw honey

1/2 c. carob powder

2 tsp. cinnamon

1 tsp. nutmeg

2 pinches sea salt

1/2 c. dried shredded coconut

> Combine all ingredients except coconut in a large bowl and mix thoroughly.

> Form into balls and roll in coconut flakes.

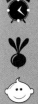

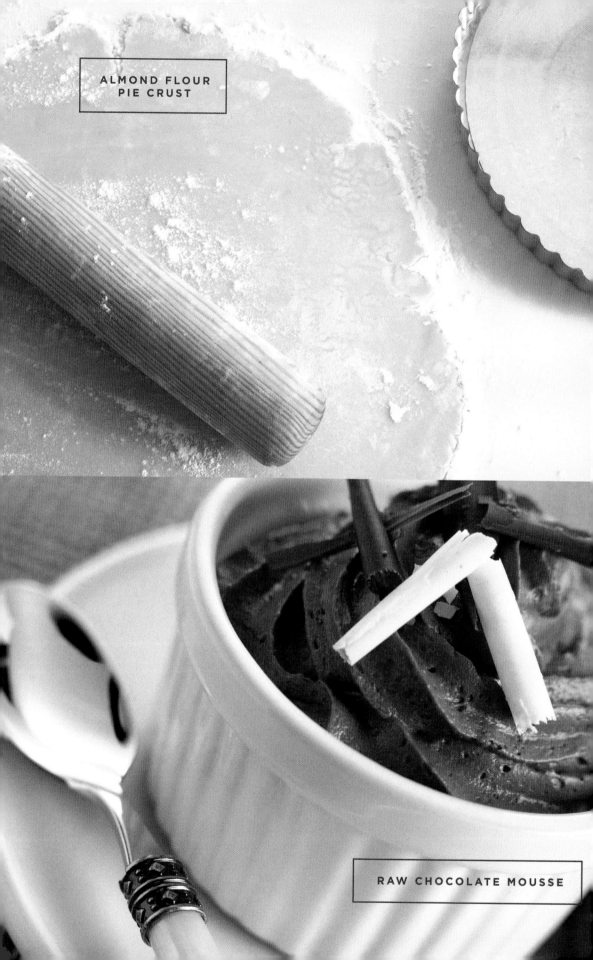

ALMOND FLOUR
PIE CRUST

RAW CHOCOLATE MOUSSE

Almond Flour Pie Crust

2 c. almond flour

1 c. rice flour

1/4 tsp. baking soda

1/4 tsp. sea salt

4 Tbsp. unsalted butter, cold, cut into small pieces

2 Tbsp. honey

1 egg

> Combine all ingredients in a food processor or powerful blender. The butter will show in the dough.

> Separate dough into 2 balls. Wrap one in wax paper and place in refrigerator.

> Place the other ball on parchment paper and roll out to fit 8 or 9 inch pie plate. Repeat with second ball of dough.

> Bake 15 minutes at 350 degrees or until browned.

Raw Chocolate Mousse

1/2 c. medjool dates, soaked

1/2 c. maple syrup

1 tsp. vanilla extract

1-1 1/2 c. mashed avocado (abt. 3 avocados)

3/4 c. organic cocoa or carob powder

1/2 c. water

> Blend or process dates, maple syrup and vanilla until smooth. Add mashed avocado and cocoa powder. Add water and process until smooth.

> Serve at room temperature or chilled.

Make fudgesicles by freezing the mousse in ice cube trays. Make chocolate sauce or fondue by increasing water to 1 c.

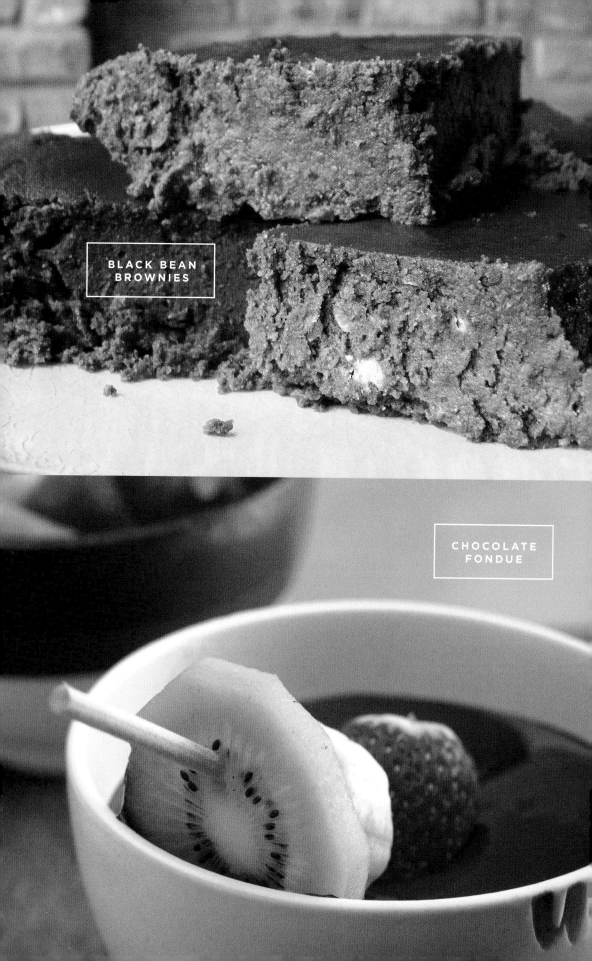

BLACK BEAN
BROWNIES

CHOCOLATE
FONDUE

Black Bean Brownies

1 15 oz. can black beans

1/2 c. cocoa

4 Tbsp. coconut oil

1/2 c. xylitol

2 tsp. stevia powder

1 tsp. vanilla

3 eggs

1/2 c. gluten free flour

1/4 tsp. sea salt

1/4 c. water

> Strain all liquid from black beans

> Place all ingredients in a blender and blend until smooth.

> Grease an 8x8 pan with coconut oil and pour batter into pan. Bake for 45 minutes at 350 degrees.

Chocolate Fondue

1 bar dark chocolate (at least 70% cocoa)

1/2 c. coconut milk

stevia to taste

> Warm coconut milk in a saucepan over medium heat. Break chocolate bar into pieces and stir into coconut milk.

> Add stevia until desired sweetness is achieved.

> Dip berries or other fruit into chocolate fondue.

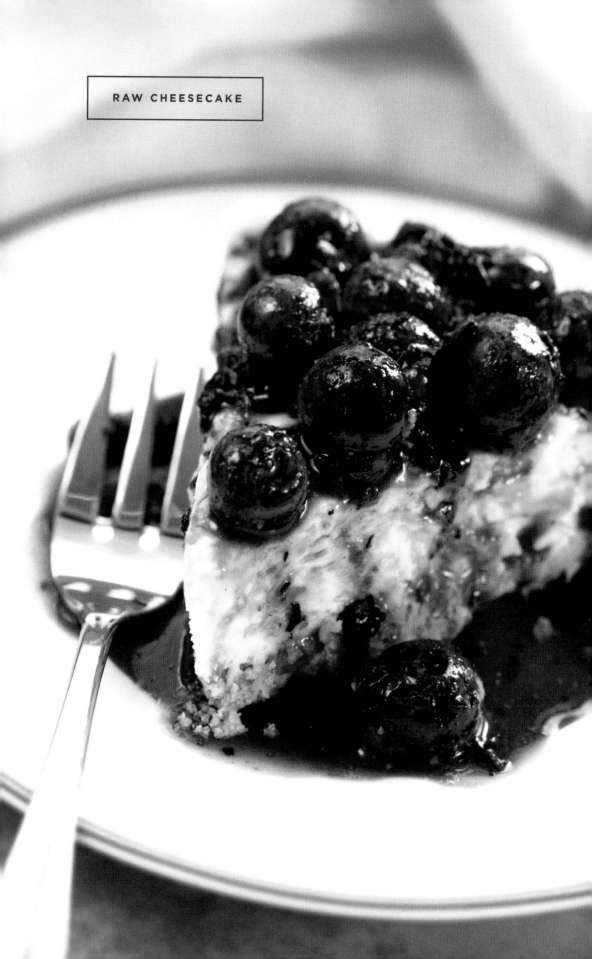

Raw Cheesecake

Crust:

2 c. raw nuts (almonds, pecans, walnuts or macadamia nuts)

1/2 c. soaked dates

coconut flakes

> Sprinkle coconut flakes on the bottom of an 8" springform pan to prevent sticking.

> Using a food processor or powerful blender, process the nuts and dates. Gently press mixture onto sides and bottom of the pan as the crust.

Filling:

3 c. soaked cashews

3/4 c. lemon juice with pulp (add lime for extra tartness)

3/4 c. raw honey

3/4 c. raw coconut oil (slightly melted)

1/4" piece vanilla bean (use scraped out seeds only)

> Using a powerful blender, blend all ingredients until smooth.

> Pour into pan and place in freezer.

Topping:

bag of frozen fruit (your choice)

dates (to taste)

> Blend a bag of your favorite frozen fruit until it is spreadable (but not smooth). Add dates to the mixture as needed for sweetness.

> Pour over cheesecake after it has set. Cover and return to the freezer.

> Defrost in refrigerator one hour before serving.

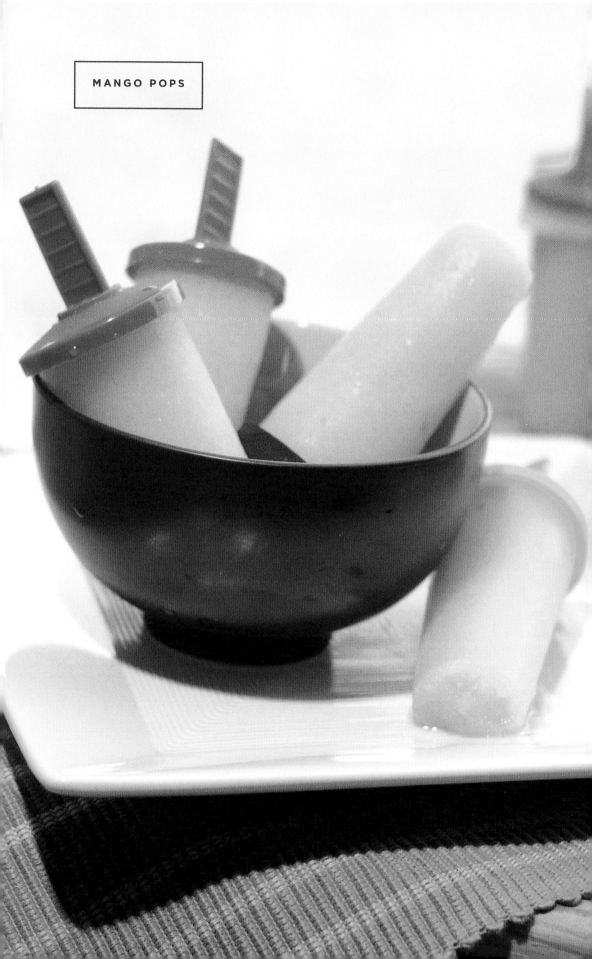

Mango Pops

4 oz. water

1/8 c. lime juice

1-2 packets stevia

1 c. mango chunks

1 c. pineapple chunks

2 c. ice cubes

> Place all ingredients in a blender and blend until smooth.

> Pour into ice cube trays or popsicle molds and place in freezer. When mixture is partially set, add a toothpick or popsicle stick for a handle.

Jesse's Dark Chocolate Milkshake

6 large ice cubes

1 c. coconut milk

2 Tbsp. raw honey

1/2 tsp. stevia

4 Tbsp. unsweetened dark cocoa powder

pinch of cinnamon (to taste)

> Place all ingredients in blender and blend until frothy.

> Serve in a chilled glass.

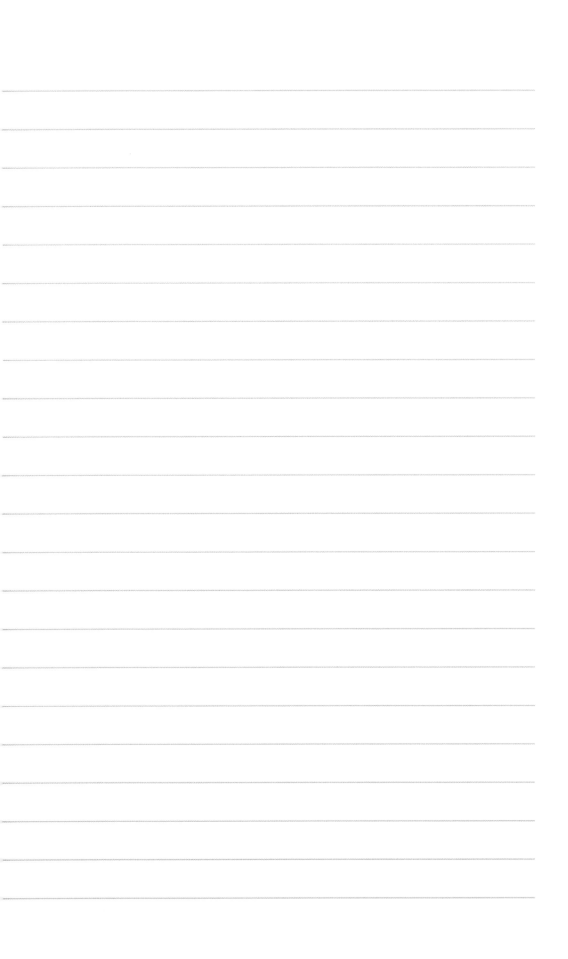